Nutrition and HIV/AIDS - Implication for Treatment, Prevention and Cure

Edited by Nancy Dumais

Published in London, United Kingdom

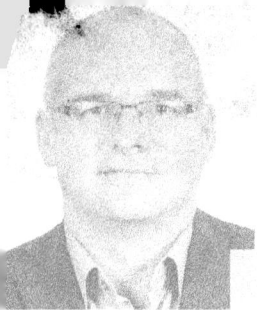
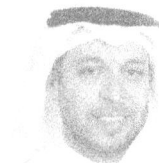
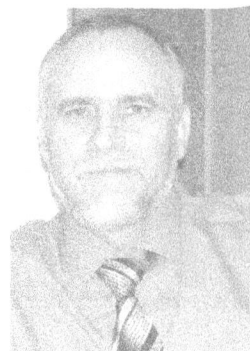
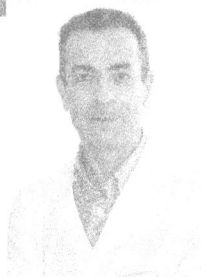
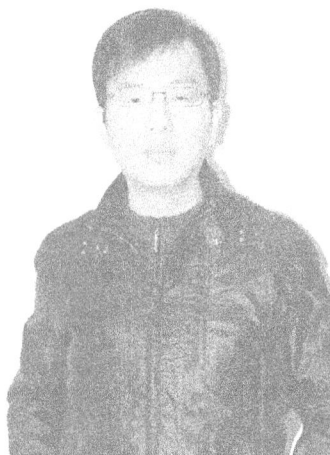
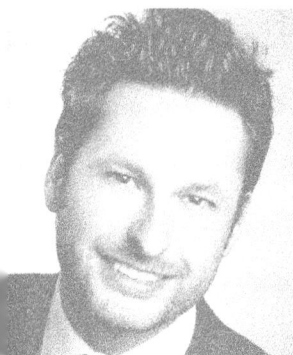
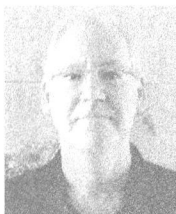

IntechOpen

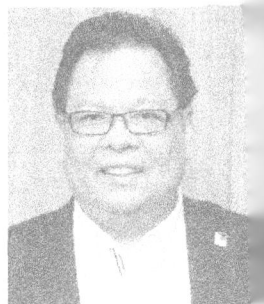
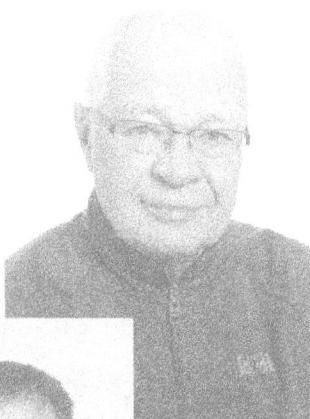
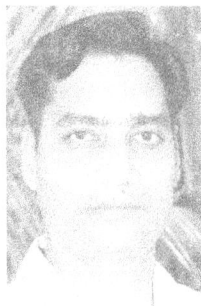
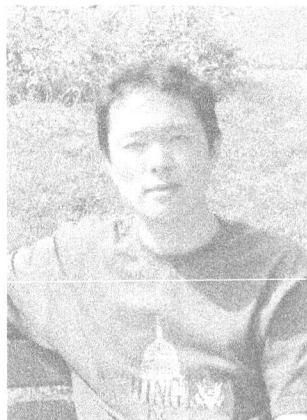
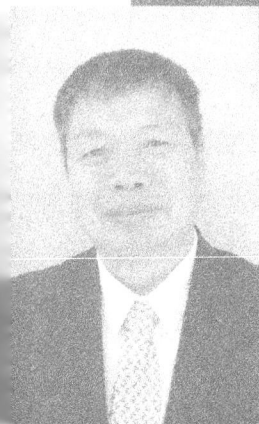
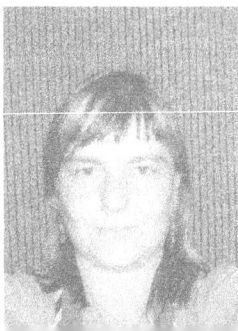

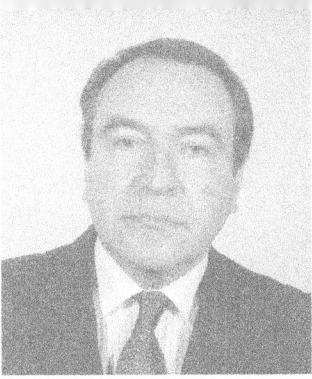

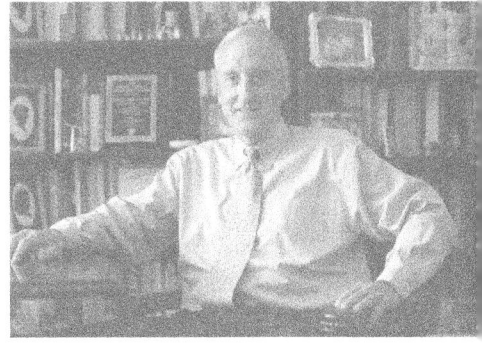

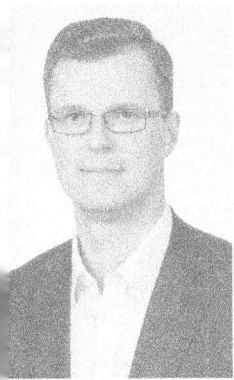

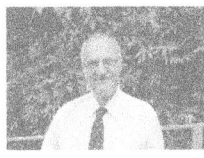

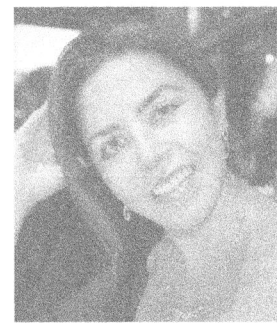

Supporting open minds since 2005

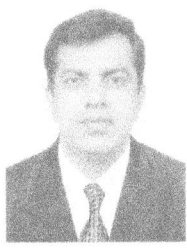

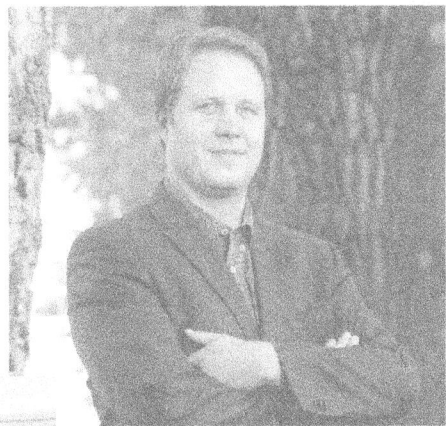

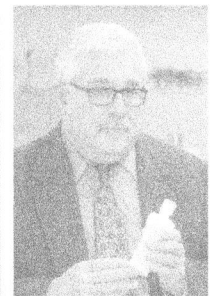

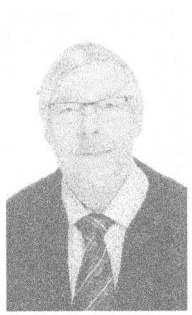

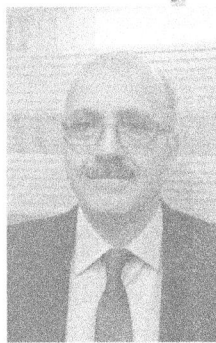

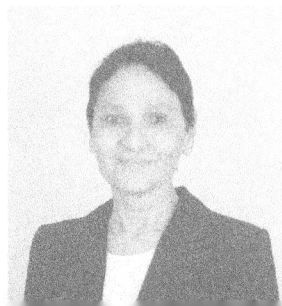

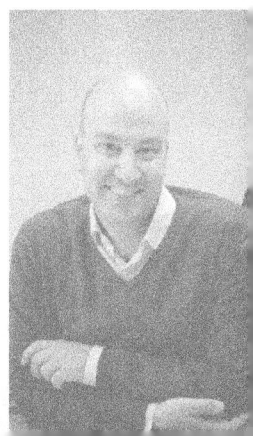

Nutrition and HIV/AIDS - Implication for Treatment, Prevention and Cure
http://dx.doi.org/10.5772/intechopen.77674
Edited by Nancy Dumais

Contributors
Negussie Boti Sidemo, Sultan Hussen, Inaya Hajj Hussein, Virginia Uhley, Abdo Jurjus, Lara Youssef, Andrea Mladenovic, Angelo Leone, V K Sashindran, Maria Dimitrova, Guenka Petrova, Ezinne Ezinna Enwereji, Martina Chikodi Ezeama, Prince Ezenwa Onyemachi

Notice
Statements and opinions expressed in the chapters are these of the individual contributors and not necessarily those of the editors or publisher. No responsibility is accepted for the accuracy of information contained in the published chapters. The publisher assumes no responsibility for any damage or injury to persons or property arising out of the use of any materials, instructions, methods or ideas contained in the book.

First published in London, United Kingdom, 2020 by IntechOpen
IntechOpen is the global imprint of INTECHOPEN LIMITED, registered in England and Wales, registration number: 11086078, 7th floor, 10 Lower Thames Street, London,
EC3R 6AF, United Kingdom
Printed in Croatia

British Library Cataloguing-in-Publication Data
A catalogue record for this book is available from the British Library

Additional hard and PDF copies can be obtained from orders@intechopen.com

Nutrition and HIV/AIDS - Implication for Treatment, Prevention and Cure
Edited by Nancy Dumais
p. cm.
Print ISBN 978-1-78984-137-4
Online ISBN 978-1-78984-138-1
eBook (PDF) ISBN 978-1-78985-061-1

We are IntechOpen,
the world's leading publisher of
Open Access books
Built by scientists, for scientists

4,800+
Open access books available

122,000+
International authors and editors

135M+
Downloads

Our authors are among the

151
Countries delivered to

Top 1%
most cited scientists

12.2%
Contributors from top 500 universities

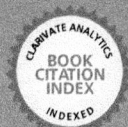

Interested in publishing with us?
Contact book.department@intechopen.com

Numbers displayed above are based on latest data collected.
For more information visit www.intechopen.com

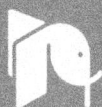

Meet the editor

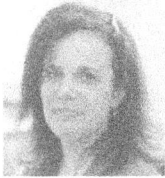

Dr Nancy Dumais is a Professor of Virology at the Université de Sherbrooke, Canada. She received her Diploma (M.Sc.) in Cellular and Molecular Biology and her Doctorate (Ph.D.) in Virology, in 1996 and 2001, respectively, both from the Université Laval in Canada. Thereafter, she was a Postdoctoral Researcher at McMaster University where she studied mucosal immunization against HIV. Her research interests include chemokines and chemokine receptors in HIV-1 pathogenesis and cell migration. Her laboratory also investigates the roles of prostaglandins in HIV transcription and replication. Also, she is interested in scientific and health education. She gives lectures in molecular biology, microbiology, and virology at different universities.

Contents

Preface

This edited volume is a collection of reviewed and relevant research chapters, concerning the developments within the "Nutrition and HIV/AIDS - Implication for Treatment, Prevention and Cure" field of study. The book includes scholarly contributions by various authors and has been edited by an expert in the field. Each contribution comes as a separate chapter complete in itself but directly related to the book's topics and objectives.

The book includes chapters dealing with the following topics: nutritional status and its effect on treatment outcome among HIV-infected children receiving first-line antiretroviral therapy in Arba Minch General Hospital and Arba Minch Health Center, Gamo Zone, Southern Ethiopia: Retrospective Cohort Study; HIV-infected children and nutrition: the friend and the foe; malnutrition in HIV/AIDS: aetio-pathogenesis; nutrition habits in people living with HIV/AIDS in Bulgaria: review of current practice and recommendations; basic principles of nutrition, HIV and AIDS: making improvements in diet to enhance health.

The target audience comprises scholars and specialists in the field.

IntechOpen

Chapter 1

Nutritional Status and Its Effect on Treatment Outcome among HIV-Infected Children Receiving First-Line Antiretroviral Therapy in Arba Minch General Hospital and Arba Minch Health Center, Gamo Zone, Southern Ethiopia: Retrospective Cohort Study

Negussie Boti Sidemo and Sultan Hussen Hebo

Abstract

Antiretroviral therapy is a drug treatment that plays a great role in reduction of mortality among children infected with human immunodeficiency virus (HIV). Studies in Africa have shown that there is short survival time among children receiving antiretroviral therapy. The aims of this study were to estimate the survival time and identify associated factors among HIV-infected children after initiation of antiretroviral therapy. Institution-based retrospective cohort study was conducted among 421 children. Cox proportional hazards regression model was used to determine independent predictors. Findings of this study reveal that 261 (62%) children were alive, 43 (10.2%) were lost to follow-up, 52 (12.4%) were transferred out to other facilities, and 65 (15.4%) were reported to have died, and overall prevalence of malnutrition among respondents was 23.7% (95% CI, 19.13–28.27%). Multivariable analysis showed that nutritional status (adjusted hazard ratio (AHR) = 4.1, 95% CI = 2.41–6.9), absolute CD4 count below threshold (AHR = 2.3, 95% CI = 1.32–3.88), fair and poor adherence to antiretroviral therapy (AHR = 0.4, 95% CI = 1.66–6.9), (AHR = 3.3, 95% CI = 1.73–6.23), isoniazid prophylaxis (AHR = 0.4, 95%, CI = 0.21–0.65), and co-trimoxazole prophylaxis (AHR = 0.3, 95% CI = 0.14–0.44) were independent predictors of the survival time. Therefore, children living with HIV should be encouraged to adhere to the antiretroviral therapy and take co-trimoxazole and isoniazid preventive therapies.

Keywords: antiretroviral therapy, co-trimoxazole preventive therapy, isoniazid preventive therapy, children, Ethiopia

1. Introduction

Acquired immune deficiency syndrome (AIDS) is a disease caused by a retro-virus known as human immunodeficiency virus (HIV) [1]. HIV/AIDS remains one of the world's most significant public health challenges, particularly in low- and middle-income countries [2]. Children constitute a segment of the population affected by the virus. HIV contributes to illness and death of children and is the commonest cause for pediatric hospital admission [3].

Of the total 1.8 million children living with HIV, an estimated 110,000 die of AIDS-related illnesses each year which means 290 children die of AIDS-related illnesses every day. Nearly 90% of HIV-infected children live in sub-Saharan Africa (SSA) [4]. In Ethiopia it is estimated that 65,088 children are living with HIV. In 2016, over 3100 children died due to AIDS-related illness [5].

The introduction of antiretroviral therapy (ART) presented an enormous opportunity in terms of reducing morbidity and mortality due to AIDS, worldwide. Ethiopia has been engaged in the scale-up of ART access to its people since 2005 [6]. It has been shown that the improvement in access to ART improves the quality of life and survival of children [7, 8].

Studies show that early access to ART could prevent 25% of HIV-related deaths [7–9]. Therefore, to reduce child mortality attributed to HIV/AIDS, the provision of comprehensive treatment, care, and support for HIV-infected children is very important.

Ethiopia has adopted the World Health Organization's (WHO) recommendations for ART where "regardless of their CD4 cell count, all HIV-infected individuals should start treatment to reduce morbidity and mortality associated with HIV infection" [3]. The number of sites providing ART service in Ethiopia, including both public and private facilities, has increased from 3 to over 1000, and persons initiated on treatment has increased from 24,000 to 308,000 during the period 2006–2016 with more than 23,400 children under the age of 15 taking antiretroviral drugs [10].

Survival of HIV-positive children in Ethiopia and other similar settings has improved as a result of increased access to ART; however, it is still low in the first 6 months after initiation of ART [11]. Reports from Kenya, Zambia, and Malawi show that death among HIV-positive children following ART initiation remains high, ranging from 7.5 to 15% [12–14]. This contrasts the substantially higher survival probability among HIV-positive children initiated on ART in developed countries [15]. Findings from other studies elsewhere in Africa and other low-income countries show that ART programs have resulted in decreased mortality among children on ART [16–18]. Available evidences also depicted that the survival of the children is not only affected by the care delivered by ART programs but also more fundamentally influenced by low CD4 count, advanced disease according to WHO staging, low hemoglobin (Hgb) level, and opportunistic infections (OIs) like bacterial pneumonia and tuberculosis [19–21]. However, as far as our search of the available literature has revealed, little is known about the effect of factors like viral load, nutritional status, co-trimoxazole (CTZ) preventive therapy (CPT), and isoniazid (INH) preventive therapy (IPT) on survival status of children below 15 years of age. Therefore, this study intended to estimate the survival time and identify associated factors by including viral load, nutritional status, CPT, and IPT among HIV-infected children initiated on ART in public health facilities in Arba Minch town, Southern Ethiopia.

2. Main body

2.1 Patients and methods

Study area and period: We conducted the study in Arba Minch town from March 20, 2017 to April 10, 2017. Arba Minch town is located about 495 km southwest of the capital city Addis Ababa and about 275 km from Hawassa, the capital of the Southern Nations, Nationalities, and Peoples' Region (SNNPR). Arba Minch town has one general hospital and one public health center, which provide ART service. Arba Minch Hospital was among the first few public hospitals to start ART in Ethiopia in August 2003. Arba Minch Health Center started ART service at the end of 2007. According to the Gamo Gofa Zone Health Department (ZHD) report, the Arba Minch Hospital and Arba Minch Health Center provide HIV/AIDS interventions, including free diagnostic, treatment, and monitoring services. Since August 2003, ART has been provided to children living with HIV regardless of CD4 count and WHO clinical stage, with financial support from the Norwegian Lutheran Mission. Data from ZHD show that a total of 664 children with HIV/AIDS were enrolled on chronic HIV care at the hospital and the health center since January 2009, but only 608 started ART (460 children at Arba Minch General Hospital and 148 children at Arba Minch Health Center) [22].

Study design: A health facility-based retrospective cohort study.

Source populations: All children living with HIV who were enrolled on first-line ART at the center.

Study populations: All children living with HIV who were enrolled on first-line ART at the center and who fulfill the inclusion criteria.

Inclusion criteria: Those who were aged <18 years and enrolled on first-line ART and have follow-up at Arba Minch General Hospital and Health Center.

Sample size determination: The sample size was calculated by applying a two-population proportion formula using Epi-Info version 7. Co-trimoxazole preventive therapy, tuberculosis (TB) co-infection at baseline, and anemia were considered, and taking the most significant predictors of the three variables, anemia was used [17] with the following assumptions: 95% CI, power 80%, ratio of unexposed to exposed 1:1, parameter outcome in exposed hemoglobin (Hgb) < 10 gm/dl = 14.7%, outcome in unexposed Hgb ≥ 10 gm/dl = 5.8%, and hazard ratio (HR) = 2.5. This resulted in sample size of 412 children. As there were a total of 421 children in the study area who fulfilled the inclusion criteria, we included all 421 in this study.

Sampling procedure and sampling technique: A total of 608 children who started ART during the study period were identified in the two ART clinics. Charts were organized according to the hospital card number, in a chronological order, with each chart representing one child. As some of the charts in the hospital were not arranged in numerical order, the investigator assigned new numbers for all those registered between 2009 and 2016, starting from 1 to 608. Of these, the investigator drew 421 samples which fulfilled the inclusion criteria after reviewing the information transcribed to the pre-structured data abstraction form; 187 individuals did not fulfill the inclusion criteria; therefore, those charts were excluded from the study. Children ≤14 years of age and on ART registered for chronic care at public health institutions of Arba Minch town from 1 January 2009 to 30 December 2016 were included in the study. Those whose cards were incomplete with information on baseline CD4 count, WHICH staging and date of ART start and current status were excluded from the study.

2.2 Variables in the study

Dependent variable: The response (outcome) variable in this study was "survival time" of HIV-infected children after starting ART.

Independent variables: The predictor variables included five continuous covariates (age, hemoglobin level, weight, height, and CD4 count) and nine categorical variables (gender, co-trimoxazole prophylaxis, TB co-infection status, isoniazid prophylaxis, functional status, clinical stage of the disease according to WHO scaling, type of ART drug, adherence to ART, and year of ART initiation).

2.3 Operational definition of terms

Censored: includes lost to follow-up, transfer out, and live beyond the study time.

Adherence to ART: assessed by counting the number of tablets the children miss within the first 3 months after starting ART.

Survival: absence of experience of death.

Survival time: the length of time in months a child was followed up from the time the child started ART until death, was lost to follow-up, or was still on follow-up.

3. Data collection procedure and data quality control

A structured interviewer-administered questionnaire was used to collect the data [23–25]. The questionnaire was primarily developed in English and then translated into Amharic language for simplicity of data collection. Then Amharic version was also back-translated to English language for its consistency by two different language experts. The data collection tool has four sections. Pretesting of the data collection tool was done on 17 individuals who were selected from Berber Health Center that were not included in the actual study. Based on the pretest, a data collection tool was corrected to ensure logical sequence, clarity, and skipping patterns. Data was collected by eight trained health professionals and supervised by two bachelor degree health professionals. All data collectors and supervisors were trained for 2 days and performed practical exercises to be familiar with the questionnaire. Exit interview was done. The participants' weight was measured in kilograms with 0.2 kg increments using standard beam balance, and the scale was checked at zero during measurement. The study participant was removing their heavy outer clothes and shoes. The participant height was measured using the standard measuring scale to the nearest 0.5 cm. The participants were asked to take off their shoes, stand erect, and look straight in vertical plain. The data collectors were regularly supervised for proper data collection as well as checked for completeness and consistency throughout data collection period.

Data processing and analysis: The completeness and consistency of the data was checked, coded, and double entered into Epi-info version 7 and exported to Statistical Package for Social Sciences (SPSS) version 20 for analysis. Exploratory data analysis was carried out to check the levels of missing values and presence of influential outliers. Descriptive statistics such as mean (standard deviation), frequencies, and proportions were used to describe the characteristics of the cohort. Kaplan-Meier survival curve together with log-rank test was used to assess survival experience of an individual at specific times and to compare survival between different independent variables.

The analysis was conducted in several steps. First, univariate Cox proportional hazard regression model was performed for each independent variable and outcome of interest to identify potentially significant variables for consideration in the multivariable Cox proportional hazards regression model. Based on the univariate analysis, variables were selected for the multivariable analysis. Variables whose univariate significance test results were below p-value <0.25 were included in the multivariable regression model. In addition, context and findings of previous studies were considered in the identification of candidate variables for multivariable analysis.

Multivariable analysis was started with a model containing all of the selected variables. The model was built through a stepwise regression procedure, which added variables successively (the most significant at each step) until no variable added significant information and compared by likelihood ratio test and Harrell's concordance statistic test. Interactions and confounders were tested and the cutoff point of beta change greater than 20% was used. The results of the final model were expressed in terms of hazard ratio with 95% confidence intervals (CI) and interpreted accordingly. Kaplan-Meier survival curve together with log-rank test was used to check for the existence of any significant differences in survival between the various categories of variables considered in this study. Statistical significance was declared if the p-value was less than 0.05.

Ethical considerations: Ethical approval was obtained from the ethical review committee of Arba Minch University, College of Medicine and Health Sciences, with reference number CMHS/4268/09. Following the approval, an official letter of cooperation was written to concerned bodies by the Department of Public Health of Arba Minch University. Permission was granted from the Hospital and Health Center Administration as per the recommendation letter from the department. Personal identifiers were excluded during data extraction; rather codes were used. Considering the study was being conducted on secondary data, obtaining informed consents from the participants was not possible. However, the confidentiality of information was maintained by not recording their name from the chart, and the recorded data were not accessed by a third person except by the principal investigator.

4. Results

Baseline characteristics of the study participant: A total of 421 study participants (children under 15 years old) were included in the study. The sample is comprised of 241 (57.2%) males and 180 (42.8%) females. The ages of the cohort at ART initiation ranged from 3 to 168 months with a median age of 72 (IQR = 33–108) months. Based on WHO clinical staging, 196 (47%) children initiated ART at an advanced stage of the disease, i.e., WHO clinical stage III or IV. During the ART initiation, 139 (33%) children were affected by one or more opportunistic illness, of which 41 children were found to have died at the end of the study. Sixty (14.3%) had history of TB at the start of ART, and 36 died during the follow-up time. At the initiation of ART, mean (SD) value for weight of children was 18.6 (±9.65) kg, and mean (SD) value for height of the cohort was 110.8 (±32.19) cm. The baseline median value for Hgb was 10.9 (IQR = 8.8–12.3) g/dl, and 181 (43.1%) of the children had absolute CD4 count below threshold for immune deficiency at initiation of ART.

Among the reviewed participants, 410 (97.4%) were on first-line ART regimen, while the rest were started on second line. Concerning the type of ART regimens, around 61% of children were taking D4T-based drug regimens when they started the treatment (**Table 1**).

Variables	Categories	Frequency	Percent
Sex	Male	241	57.2
	Female	180	42.8
Age category	<1 year	30	7.1
	1–4 years	169	40.1
	5–14 years	222	52.7
Primary caregiver	Parents	268	63.7
	Relatives	119	28.3
	Guardian/orphan	34	8.0
Parental status	Both parents are alive	260	61.8
	Maternal orphan	45	10.9
	Paternal orphan	31	7.4
	Double orphan	84	19.9
WHO clinical staging at entry	Stage I	91	21.6
	Stage II	135	32.1
	Stage III	147	34.9
	Stage IV	48	11.4
TB at baseline	Yes	60	14.3
	No	361	85.7
Hemoglobin level at baseline	<10 gm/dl	78	18.5
	≥10 gm/dl	343	81.5
Absolute CD4 at baseline	CD4 above threshold	239	56.9
	CD4 below threshold	181	43.1
ART adherence status	Good	335	79.6
	Fair	33	7.8
	Poor	53	12.6
CTZ prophylaxis	Yes	314	74.6
	No	107	25.4
INH prophylaxis	Yes	302	71.7
	No	119	28.3

Table 1.
Demographic and clinical characteristics and chemoprophylaxis status among children on antiretroviral treatment at Arba Minch Hospital and Health Center, Southern Ethiopia, 2017.

5. Mean survival time after initiation of ART

After initiation of ART, children were followed up for a minimum of 1 and maximum of 95 months with median follow-up period of 50 (IQR = 24–80) months. At the end of follow-up, 261 (62%) of the children were alive, 43 (10.2%) were lost to follow-up, 52 (12.4%) were transferred out to other facilities, and 65 (15.4%) were reported dead. The overall mean estimated survival time after ART initiation of children in the study was 82.3 (95% CI = 79.48–85.14) months.

There is a significantly different survival time between different factors considered in this study. Females have relatively lower survival time of 79.3 months than males with 84.6 months. Children 1–4 years of age had higher survival time of 86.8 months than those less than 1 and 5–14 years of age who had a mean survival time of 69.3 and 80.8 months, respectively.

6. Comparison of survival curves

The overall Kaplan-Meier survivor function estimate showed that most of the deaths occurred in the earlier months of ART initiation, which declined in the later months of follow-up. Most of the graphs did not show differences between different categories. However, relatively larger gaps are observed in covariates such as WHO clinical stage, TB co-infection, low Hgb level (<10gm/dl), and CTZ and INH prophylaxes (**Figures 1** and **2**).

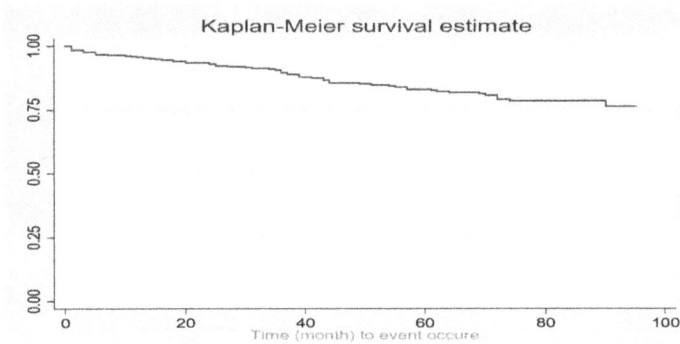

Figure 1.
The plot of the overall estimate of Kaplan-Meier survivor function among children on ART at public health facilities of Arba Minch town, Southern Ethiopia, 2017.

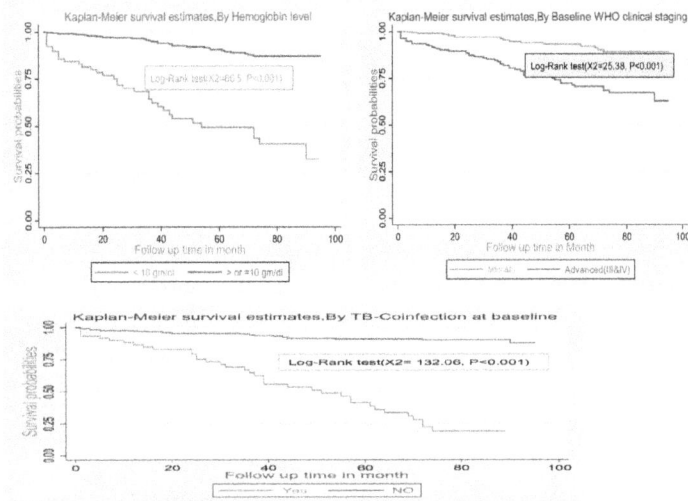

Figure 2.
Survival curves for children on ART by WHO clinical stage, hemoglobin level, and TB co-infection after start on ART at public health facilities in Arba Minch town, 2017.

7. Results of the Cox proportional hazards regression model

One important predictor of low survival time in univariable Cox regression analysis was advanced WHO staging. The risk of low survival chance in individuals with advanced disease according to WHO staging at baseline was nearly 4 times

Covariate/factor	Categories	CHR	P-values
Sex	Male		
	Female	1.617	0.053*
Age group	<1 year		
	1–4 years	1.259	0.336
	5–14 years	0.655	0.069*
Nutritional status	Normal		
	Underweight	1.903	0.010*
Anemia	No		
	Yes	2.702	0.001*
Absolute CD4 count	Above threshold		
	Below threshold	1.293	0.041*
INH prophylaxis	No		
	Yes	0.408	0.001*
CTZ prophylaxis	No		
	Yes	0.348	0.001*
ART adherence on follow-up	Good		
	Fair	6.256	0.001*
	Poor	5.937	0.001*
WHO clinical staging at entry	Stage I and II		
	Stage III	2.360	0.009*
	Stage IV	10.412	0.001*
Functional status	Working		
	Ambulatory	1.302	0.350
	Bedridden	1.375	0.392
ART regimens at entry	D4t-based regimen	0.294	0.420
	AZT-based regimen	0.513	0.290
	TDF-based regimen	0.562	0.404
	Second-line ART		
Evidence of TB during follow-up	Yes	1.383	0.050*
	No		

*Note: CTZ, Cotrimoxazole; ART, antiretroviral therapy; INH, isoniazid; TB, tuberculosis; OI, opportunistic Infections, *p < 0.25 which are candidate for Multivariate Cox regression model.*

Table 2.
Univariable Cox regression analysis of sociodemographic characteristics and clinical and immunological status among children who were started on ART at public health facilities of Arba Minch town, 2017.

higher than that of those at the mild stage of the disease (P < 0.001). The risk of surviving a shorter time in individuals who had severe acute malnutrition (SAM) at baseline was nearly 2.5 times higher when compared to those with no malnutrition (P < 0.006). Patients with baseline opportunistic infections (OIs) survive nearly three 3 times shorter than those without OIs (P < 0.001), and children with TB co-infection were nearly 11 times more likely to survive shorter when compared to those without TB co-infection (P < 0.001). The risk of surviving at short duration was significantly higher with low hemoglobin level (CHR = 7.3, 95% CI = 4.47–11.9,

Covariate	Categories	AHR	P-values
Nutritional status	Normal	1	
	Underweight	4.08	0.001
Absolute CD4 count	Above threshold	1	
	Below threshold	2.26	0.003
INH prophylaxis	No	1	
	Yes	0.37	0.001
CTZ prophylaxis	No	1	
	Yes	0.25	0.001
ART adherence on follow-up	Good	1	
	Fair	3.39	0.001
	Poor	3.28	0.001

Table 3.
Multivariable Cox regression analysis of sociodemographic characteristics and clinical and immunological status among children on ART at public health facilities of Arba Minch town, 2017.

P = 0.001) and CD4 count below the threshold (CHR = 1.7, 95% CI = 1.02–2.74, P = 0.041) when starting ART compared to their counterparts. CTZ and INH had preventive effect against surviving for short duration (CHR = 0.2, 95% CI = 0.10– 0.27 P = 0.001) and (CHR = 0.1, 95% CI = 0.07–0.20 P = 0.001) when compared to their counterparts throughout the follow-up period, respectively (**Table 2**).

In multivariable Cox regression analysis, children with CD4 count below threshold for immunodeficiency at ART initiation were 2.3 times (AHR = 2.26, 95% CI = 1.32–3.88, P = 0.003) more likely to survive at shorter duration as compared to those with CD4 count above threshold. Children with low weight for age (under-weight) at ART initiation were almost 4 times (AHR = 4.1, 95% CI = 2.41–6.9, P = 0.001) more likely to survive at shorter duration as compared to those with normal weight. Children that were presented for treatment with fair ART adherence and poor ART adherence were on follow-up 3.4 times (AHR = 3.4, 95% CI = 1.66– 6.9, P = 0.001) and 3.3 times (AHR = 3.3, 95% CI = 1.73–6.23, P = 0.001) and more likely to survive at shorter duration, respectively, as compared to those with good adherence on follow-up. Estimated AHR for children on INH prophylaxis and CTZ prophylaxis were 0.4 (95% CI = 0.21–0.65, P = 0.001) and 0.3 (95% CI = 0.14–0.44, P = 0.001); short duration survival hazard among children who took INH prophy-laxis was 63% and CTZ prophylaxis 75% (**Table 3**).

8. Discussion

In this study the overall mean survival time was 82.3 months (95% CI: 79.48– 85.14). The cumulative probability of survival of children on ART was 82.9% after 5 years (95% CI: 78.2%–86.7%). The major factors that affect the survival time of children with HIV/AIDS and on ART are nutritional status, absolute CD4 count below threshold, and poor/fair adherence to ART. Isoniazid prophylaxis and co-trimoxazole prophylaxis were preventive factors.

Mean survival time in our cohort was 82.3 months (95% CI = 79.48–85.14). This was in line with the finding of a study conducted in Southwest Ethiopia [83 months (95% CI = 79–87)] [26]. However, our finding was higher when com-pared with study conducted in Northwest Ethiopia, which reported a survival time of 56.5 months [20]. This difference might be associated with the high proportion (74.3%) of children in this study taking CTZ prophylaxis as compared to the finding of the study conducted in Northwest Ethiopia (52.3–70.4%), and the difference might also be associated with increased access to ART services.

The cumulative probability of survival of children on ART in our study was 82.9% after 5 years (95% CI: 78.2–86.7%). This was comparable with the report of a study conducted in Felege Hiwot Referral Hospital, Bahir Dar, Northern Ethiopia (83%) [27] and another one in Northwest Ethiopia (83%) [20]. However the cumulative survival probability from our study was much lower than that of the reports from Adama Referral Hospital and Medical College, Central Ethiopia (91.6%) [19], and Wolaita zone health facilities, Southern Ethiopia (92%) [20]. These variations between our study and those from central and Southern Ethiopia may have something to do with the variation in the quality of care provided at different institutions.

In this study we found that having CD4 cell count below the threshold level was significantly associated with an increased probability of having short duration of survival among the children. This concurs with the findings of different studies previously done in Ethiopia [20, 28]. The similarity might be related to the fact that children, in our series, with absolute CD4 counts below the threshold level are more prone to OIs like TB. Another possible explanation could be ART was initiated in an advanced HIV stage (stages III and IV) where immunity of the children was already compromised.

Another covariate that had a significant effect on survival time was adherence to ART. The HR for poor adherence was 2.1 times, and the HR for fair adherence was 2.2 times more likely to result in short duration of survival compared to children with good adherence. This finding was supported by studies conducted in Northwest Ethiopia [28] and Wolaita zone health facilities [20]. The poor adherence might be due to insufficient counseling and education of caregiver/patient.

The initiation of CTZ and INH at the start of ART in our cohort was associated with a longer duration of survival. This finding concurred with that of the studies conducted in Felege Hiwot Referral Hospital, Northern Ethiopia [20], and rural Mozambique [29]. The possible reason for higher risk of shorter survival time among children who did not receive CTZ at ART initiation could be due to occurrence of OIs such as *Pneumocystis pneumonia*, toxoplasmosis, bacterial pneumonia, sepsis, and diarrhea. Co-trimoxazole prophylaxis should be given at the initiation of ART to reduce OI and associated short duration survival among HIV-positive children on ART, thereby improving their survival.

The hazards of short survival time for children on INH prophylaxis was 0.38, which means that, in those children who take INH prophylaxis, the hazard of short duration of survival was reduced by 62%. This finding corroborates the finding of the study conducted in Mizan-Aman General Hospital, in Southern Ethiopia [26], and that of a double blinded, placebo-controlled trial on INH efficacy among HIV children infected in Cape Town, South Africa [30]. A possible reason could be INH prophylactic therapy (IPT) prevented the occurrence of TB.

There are some strengths and limitations of this study. The strengths of this study are the use of standard measurements which enabled to make the comparison of findings with other national and international literatures to be valid. In addition, considering long duration of follow-up period of children on ART and the inclusion of important predictors like CTZ, INH and nutritional status also add to the strength to this study. Since our study is retrospective based on available records, excluding those with incomplete information, survival time might be underestimated.

9. Conclusion

In general, this study showed that the probability of survival of children on ART was 73.9% after 96 months and the overall mean survival time was 82.3 months.

The main independent predictors of the survival time were nutritional status, absolute CD4 count below threshold, poor/fair adherence to ART, and absence of INH prophylaxis and CTZ prophylaxis. However, sex, age, advanced disease according to WHO clinical stage, and presence of TB at baseline were not predictors of survival time. Therefore, children living with HIV should be encouraged to take prophylaxis drugs like CTZ and INH. This could be achieved by collective efforts of all concerned bodies on high-risk groups such as children with OI especially TB after initiation of ART and a careful monitoring and follow-up of the children.

Acknowledgements

We would like to say thank you very much to the health facilities administrator of the hospital and health center, health professionals, and data collectors who contributed to this work.

Competing interest

The authors declare that there was no competing interest in connection to this research and its result.

Authors' contribution

NB conceived and designed the study, developed data collection instruments, and supervised data collection. NB and SH participated in the testing and finalization of the data collection instruments and coordinated study progress. NB and SH performed the statistical analysis; SH wrote all versions of the manuscript. All authors read and approved the final manuscript.

Acronyms and abbreviations

ART	antiretroviral therapy
AHR	adjusted hazard rate
AIDS	acquired immune deficiency syndrome
CPT	co-trimoxazole preventive therapy
FMOH	Federal Ministry of Health
HIV	human immune virus
NNRT	nonnucleated reverse transcripts
SAM	severe acute malnutrition
UNICEF	United Nations Children's Fund
WHO	World Health Organization

Author details

Negussie Boti Sidemo* and Sultan Hussen Hebo
Department of Public Health, College of Medicine and Health Sciences,
Arba Minch University, Arba Minch, Ethiopia

*Address all correspondence to: hanehalid@gmail.com

IntechOpen

References

[1] Ethiopian Health and Nutrition Research Institute (2012). HIV/AIDS estimates and projections in Ethiopia, 2011-2016. Addis Ababa. 2012

[2] United Nations. On the Fast Track to Ending the AIDS Epidemic (2016). Report of the Secretary-General, United Nations, New York. 2016

[3] Panel on Antiretroviral Therapy and Medical Management of HIV-Infected Children. Guidelines for the Use of Antiretroviral Agents in Pediatric HIV Infection (2016). A Working Group of the Office of AIDS Research Advisory Council (OARAC); Addis Ababa. 2016

[4] United Nations Children's Fund (2016), For Every Child, End AIDS—Seventh stocktaking Report, UNICEF, New York. 2016

[5] The Ethiopian Public Health Institute (2017). HIV Related Estimates and Projections for Ethiopia–2017, Addis Ababa. 2017

[6] Seyoum E, Mekonen Y, Kassa A, Eltom A, Damtew T, Lera M, et al. ART scale-up in Ethiopia: Success and challenges: HAPCO Plan, Monitoring and Evaluation Directorate, 2009, Addis Ababa, Ethiopia. 2009

[7] Kyawswamyint MA, Moe H, Win K, Mon O. The effectiveness of 2 years of first line antiretroviral therapy among HIV-infected children at an integrated HIV-Care Clinic in Myanmar. Journal of Pediatrics & Child Care. 2015;1(1):6

[8] Collins IJ, Jourdain G, Hansudewechakul R, Kanjanavanit S, Hongsiriwon S, Ngampiyasakul C, et al. Long-term survival of HIV-infected children receiving antiretroviral therapy in Thailand: A 5-year observational cohort study. Clinical Infectious Diseases. 2010;51(12):2010

[9] Kabue MM, Buck WC, Wanless SR, Cox CM, McCollum ED, Caviness AC, et al. Mortality and clinical outcomes in HIV-infected children on antiretroviral therapy in Malawi, Lesotho, and Swaziland. American Academy of Pediatrics. Sep 2012;130(3):e591

[10] Federal HIV/AIDS. Prevention and Control Office [FHAPCO]. Country Progress Report on the HIV Response. Federal Democratic Republic of Ethiopia. Addis Ababa: FHAPCO; 2016

[11] Reddi A, Leeper SC, Grobler AC, Geddes R, France KH, et al. Preliminary outcomes of a paediatric highly active antiretroviral therapy cohort from KwaZulu-Natal, South Africa. BMC Pediatrics. Dec 2007;7(1):13

[12] Rouet F, Fassinou P, Inwoley A, Anaky MF, Kouakoussui A, et al. Long-term survival and immuno-virological response of African HIV-1-infected children to highly active antiretroviral therapy regimens. AIDS. 2006;20:2315-2319

[13] Song R, Jelagat J, Dzombo D, Mwalimu M, Mandaliya K, et al. Efficacy of highly active antiretroviral therapy in HIV-1 infected children in Kenya. Pediatrics. 2007;120:e856-e861

[14] Wamalwa DC, Farquhar C, Obimbo EM, Selig S, Mbori-Ngacha DA, et al. Early response to highly active antiretroviral therapy in HIV-1-infected Kenyan children. Journal of Acquired Immune Deficiency Syndromes. 2007;45:311-317

[15] Gibb DM, Duong T, Tookey PA, Sharland M, Tudor-Williams G, et al. Decline in mortality, AIDS, and hospital admissions in perinatally HIV-1 infected children in the United Kingdom and Ireland. BMJ. 2003;327:1019

[16] Foca M, Moye J, Matthews Y, Rich K, Luzuriaga EHK, et al. Gender differences in lymphocyte populations, plasma HIV RNA levels, and disease progression in a cohort of children born to women infected with HIV. Pediatrics. 2006;**118**:146. DOI: 10.1542/peds.2005-0294

[17] Eley B, Nuttall J, Davies MA, Smith L, Cowburn C, Buys H, et al. Initial experience of a public-sector antiretroviral treatment programme for HIV-infected children and their infected parents. South African Medical Journal. 2004;**94**(8):643-646

[18] Ellis J, Molyneux EM. Experience of antiretroviral treatment for HIV-infected children in Malawi, the 1st 12 months. Annals of Tropical Paediatrics. 2007;**27**(4):261-267

[19] Adem AK, Alem D, Girmatsion F. Factors affecting survival of HIV positive children taking antiretroviral therapy at Adama Referral Hospital and Medical College, Ethiopia. Journal of AIDS and Clinical Research. 2014;5(3)

[20] Koye DN, Ayele TA, Zeleke BM. Predictors of mortality among children on antiretroviral therapy at a referral hospital, Northwest Ethiopia: A retrospective follow up study. BMC Pediatrics. 2012;**12**:161

[21] Ebissa G, Deyessa N, Biadgilign S. Predictors of early mortality in a cohort of HIV-infected children receiving high active antiretroviral treatment in public hospitals in Ethiopia. AIDS Care. 2015;**27**(6):723-730

[22] Gamo Gofa Zone Health Department Annual Report, Arba Minch, Ethiopia. 2016

[23] Fetzer BC, Hosseinipour MC, Kamthuzi P, Hyde L, Bramson B, Jobarteh K, et al. Predictors for mortality and loss to follow-up among children receiving antiretroviral therapy in Lilongwe, Malaw. Tropical Medicine and International Health. 2010;**14**(8):2010

[24] Wamalwa DC, Obimbo EM, Farquhar C, Richardson BA, Mbori-Ngacha DA, Inwani I, et al. Predictors of mortality in HIV-1 infected children on antiretroviral therapy in Kenya: A prospective cohort. BMC Pediatrics. 2010;**10**(33):2010

[25] Sutcliffe CG, Van Dijk JH, Munsanje B, Hamangaba F, Siniwymaanzi P, Thuma PE, et al. Risk factors for pre-treatment mortality among HIV-infected children in rural Zambia: A cohort study. PLoS One. Dec 2011;**6**(12):e29294

[26] Tezera M, Demissew B, Fikire E. Survival analysis of HIV infected people on antiretroviral therapy at Mizan-Aman general hospital, Southwest Ethiopia. International Journal of Science and Research (IJSR). 2014;**3**:5

[27] Atnafu H, Wencheko E. Factors affecting the survival of HIV-infected children after ART initiation in Bahir-Dar, Ethiopia. Ethiopian Journal of Health Development. 2012;**26**(3):193-199

[28] Shimelash B, Alemayehu M, Meselech A. Assessment of the effect of malnutrition on survival of HIV infected children after initiation of antiretroviral treatment in Wolaita zone health facilities, SNNPR, Ethiopia. A thesis to be submitted to Addis Ababa university school of public health in partial fulfillment of the requirements for degree of masters of public health in Epidemiology and Biostatistics. Addis Ababa; 2014

[29] Vermund SH, Blevins M, Moon TD, Jose E, Moiane L, Tique JA, et al. Poor clinical outcomes for HIV infected children on antiretroviral therapy in rural Mozambique: Need for program quality improvement and

community engagement. PLoS One. 2014;**9**(10):e110116

[30] Frigati LJ, Kranzer K, Cotton MF, Schaaf HS, Lombard CJ, Zar HJ. The impact of isoniazid preventive therapy and antiretroviral therapy on tuberculosis in children infected with HIV in a high tuberculosis incidence setting. Thorax. 2011;**66**(6):496-501

Chapter 2

HIV-Infected Children and Nutrition: The Friend and The Foe

Inaya Hajj Hussein, Lara Youssef, Andrea Mladenovic,
Angelo Leone, Abdo Jurjus and Virginia Uhley

Abstract

The impact of nutrition on HIV-infected children has been evaluated in multiple studies. Our review of the current trends of nutrition-related studies revealed that the focus has moved from simply the disease consequences of HIV to ensuring that antiretroviral therapy-treated children are well nourished to ensure growth and development. This update aims to present the state of the art regarding nutrition of HIV-infected children and the real potential for nutrition to serve as a dynamic therapy in this group. Recent World Health Organization reports indicate that the HIV/AIDS disease is curbing in incidence worldwide despite the high 1.8 million children, less than 15 years, reported in 2017. In addition, the literature supports the complexity and bidirectional relation between nutrition and HIV. HIV infection has a substantial effect on the nutritional status, in particular, the gastrointestinal side effects, which, in turn, have a profound impact on HIV infection. Advances in the field have transformed the course of the disease into a chronic illness, where more attention was given to lifestyle and quality of life including nutrition. However, achievement of food security, nutrition accessibility, and appropriate handling of nutrition-related complications of HIV infection are remarkable challenges, particularly, in resource poor environments, where most HIV infections exist.

Keywords: HIV/AIDS, HIV-infected children, nutrition in HIV, nutrition for children, adjunct therapy for HIV

1. Introduction

Good nutrition is essential for normal growth and development of children, and it is a vital component associated with overall health. Children infected with HIV have known increased nutrient needs to maintain optimal nutrition status. In addition, the focus of nutrition interventions has moved over the past two decades, from simply supporting the patient to ensuring that the treated children are well nourished, since they have the additional nutritional demands of growth and development [1]. Related studies have also shown that nutrition is not only an adjunct therapy but potentially a primary therapy in locations with limited access to antivirals [2].

It is also well established that HIV infection has a substantial impact on nutritional status and that nutritional status has a profound effect on the course of HIV infection [3]. The gastrointestinal side effects of HIV treatments have been well described in the literature [4].

Advances in screening and treatment modalities have decreased incidence and have transformed the course of this disease into a chronic illness [4]. In this respect, more attention has been given to the quality-of-life issues such as nutrition [3]. It is important to note that the nutrition-related complications of HIV infections, especially the achievement of food and nutrition security, are remarkable challenges, particularly, in countries of poor resources, where most HIV-infections exist. In addition, children on highly active antiretroviral therapy (HAART) require higher levels of nutritional supplementation, in particular during the initiation period of the treatment [5]. To deal with such issues, a series of guidelines have been developed by WHO and professional societies. However, the adherence to such guidelines has been reported to have encountered many obstacles in different countries.

2. Epidemiology of HIV/AIDS in children

Despite the fact that the HIV/AIDS pandemic is curbing, in 2017, there were 36.9 million people living with HIV (35.1 million adults and 1.8 million children <15 years). Only 52% of children living with HIV were receiving lifelong antiretroviral therapy (ART). In addition, 940,000 people died from AIDS-related illnesses in 2017, while AIDS-related deaths have been reduced by more than 51% since the peak in 2004 [6].

It is well established that without treatment, HIV infection causes progressive immunosuppression, due to HIV virus-mediated depletion of CD4+ lymphocytes, leaving patients at risk of developing opportunistic infections and other HIV-related disorders [7, 8]. Since the mid-1990s, the introduction of highly active antiretroviral therapy (HAART) has remarkably influenced the epidemiology of pediatric HIV type 1 infection [9]. Consequently, the prognosis of HIV-infected children has markedly improved, both in terms of mortality and morbidity [9, 10].

The mother-to-child transmission (MTCT) was basically the focus for developing new and innovative strategies to prevent vertical transmission. In the absence of preventive measures, the risk of transmission is pretty significant as it ranges between 15 and 40%. Multiple factors affect the rate of MCTC transmission; they include maternal viral load and duration of exposure. The viral transfer is also enhanced in the presence of breast lesions or vaginal delivery. In western countries (USA and Europe), the MTCT has dropped to less than 1% in the last 10 years [8]. Such a decline is basically due to the implementation of new HIV management guidelines, which include (a) antenatal testing, (b) antiviral prophylaxis early in pregnancy, (c) elective cesarean delivery before labor, and (d) avoidance of breast feeding [8, 11].

Two developments have had the greatest impact on the outcome of pediatric HIV infection:

- The availability and use of highly effective, combination antiretroviral therapy (ART) and

- The early initiation of ART in HIV-infected infants [11]. Although the mortality rate in HIV-infected children is still considerably higher than the pediatric general population, it has decreased to 0.5–0.9 per 100 children per year in recent years [9].

Mortality rates in resource-limited environments were 4.5, 6.9, and 7.7% at 1, 2, and 3 years, respectively. These rates are similar to those observed among children in developed settings [12]. Despite these encouraging results and increasing access to

ART, mortality remains high for HIV-infected children in low- and middle-income countries. Risk factors for mortality in the first year of ART treatment include young age, low CD4 percent, advanced clinical disease, anemia, and low weight for age [13, 14]. In resource-limited countries, HIV can infect the most productive family members, especially parents, reducing agricultural production and the economic capacity of the household, causing insecure provision of food for children [2].

3. HIV infection and malnutrition in children

The cooccurrence of HIV and malnutrition together increases comorbidities and mortality in affected individuals [15]. Severe acute malnutrition (SAM) is of particular concern in children with HIV [1]. SAM is defined by the World Health Organization (WHO) as a weight-for-height z-score of less than −3, or a mid-upper arm circumference (MUAC) of less than 11.5 cm in children aged 6 months to 5 years. It can present as either marasmus (protein energy malnutrition nonedematous), kwashiorkor (edematous disease), or as marasmic-kwashiorkor. However, marasmus is seen more commonly in HIV-positive children. Although the prevalence of children with HIV and severe acute malnutrition (SAM) is variable, mortality from SAM is more than three times higher in HIV-positive children than HIV-negative children. In addition, they have a higher risk of infectious comorbidities and complications [15–17]. Nine out of 10 studies on HIV-infected children, conducted in countries with limited food resources, described low height for age, and all 10 studies reported poor weight gain. Such malnutrition was described under several forms:

- Chronic malnutrition: In this category, there is small height for age caused by several in utero infections. Such infections, which can also occur in early childhood, could be coupled with other deficiencies. Such malnutrition has a significant impact on the normal development of 39% or 56 million children less than 5 years [18].

- Acute malnutrition: In this form, there is low weight for height resulting from a recent infection or a deficiency, whereby vital functions are impaired, leading to more mortality. However, the situation could be reversed with the appropriate nutritional support. It affects 9% or 13 million children less than 5 years in sub-Saharan Africa [18].

- Underweight: In this group, there is also low weight for age. The child is thin, and it is hard to differentiate it from the two other groups. However, it could be considered as an indicator to follow up on the nutritional status of a child. It has been reported to impact 21% of children below 5 years of age in sub-Saharan Africa (30 million children). In brief, wide regional disparities have been reported in the prevalence of malnutrition in individuals infected with HIV. West and Central Africa are among the most impacted by underweight and acute malnutrition (22 and 11%, respectively), while the highest chronic malnutrition rates are found in East Africa 42% [18].

4. Malnutrition and the immune system

The relationship between malnutrition and HIV in children is complex. These two conditions interact and can create a vicious circle of poor health outcomes. Moreover, multiple studies have documented the positive effect of appropriate

	HIV-infected (n = 16)	HIV-negative (n = 46)	p-Value
	Mean ± SEM		
Fatty acid metabolites			
• NEFA (mmol/L)	0.65 ± 0.10	0.54 ± 0.06	0.285
• Total ketones (μmol/L)	826 ± 259	424 ± 95	**0.0387**
Acylcarnitines			
• C2 (μmol/L)	22.3 ± 3.5	14.4 ± 2.4	**0.0103**
• Even-chain acylcarnitine molar sum (μmol/L)	24.0 ± 3.7	16.0 ± 2.6	**0.0108**
Hormones			
• Insulin (μIU/ml)	1.81 ± 0.48	2.45 ± 0.45	0.321
• Growth hormone (ng/ml)	12.4 ± 2.7	11.0 ± 1.3	0.380
Adipocytokines[*]	**n = 13**	**n = 46**	
• Leptin (pg/ml)	69.8 ± 26.6	292 ± 52	**0.0163**
• Total adiponectin (ng/ml)	8049 ± 1081	15,268 ± 1133	**0.0017**
• HMW adiponectin (ng/ml)	4409 ± 757	9356 ± 761	**0.0014**
Amino acids			
• Alanine	153 ± 27.4	217 ± 16.2	**0.0330**
• Valine	100 ± 10.7	75.6 ± 6.3	**0.0248**
• Phenylalanine	79.6 ± 7.7	43.0 ± 4.5	**0.0067**
• Amino acid molar sum (μmol/L)	1230 ± 62	1190 ± 51	0.417
Inflammatory cytokines			
• IL-2 (pg/ml)	7.7 ± 2.7	3.6 ± 1.2	**0.0158**
• TNF-α (pg/ml)	43.0 ± 5.5	37.4 ± 9.5	**0.0248**
Other			
• Glucose (mg/dl)	77.1 ± 7.9	85.9 ± 3.9	0.474
• Creatinine (mg/dl)	0.30 ± 0.04	0.27 ± 0.03	0.296
• Triglycerides (mg/dl)	177.6 ± 14.0	122.9 ± 12.2	**0.0008**

Excludes patients on ARVs.
Adapted from [22].

Table 1.
Relevant baseline metabolic profile of HIV-infected and HIV-negative patients. Bold values denote statistical significance at the p<0.05 level.

nutrition of vitamins and antioxidants, cofactors of metabolic pathways, in enhancing and potentiating the immune system. On the other hand, malnutrition has also been implicated in impairing immunity, which could even lead to an immunodeficiency status with degraded lymphoid tissue containing lower concentrations of CD4 cells, target of HIV [5, 15]. In such a weak or deficient immune system, the ability to combat infections is reduced. Consequently, malnutrition can speed up the progression of the HIV/AIDS disease by creating a favorable environment, which contributes to the oxidative stress, which accelerates the death of the immune cells and increase viral replication. Stressing the necessity of vitamin A and iron, some authors associated their deficiencies with higher mortality risk among HIV/AIDS patients [19]. In fact, HIV-infected patients have, in general, an enhanced activity of proinflammatory cytokines (TNF-α, IL-1, IL-6, and others), which can cause in children among other side effects retarded growth and a loss in body weight. At the same time, such immune-compromised children will acquire opportunistic infections, which will decrease by themselves the intake of food, thus leading to the aggravation of the immunodeficiency state and the higher incidence of several overlapping infections, such as tuberculosis, oral and esophageal candidiasis, pneumonia, skin infections, and persistent diarrhea. All these complications will negatively affect the nutritional status. In addition, anemia, which is a possible consequence of malnutrition, is also a complication of HIV infection that can cause growth retardation in children [2, 15, 20]. These children often require highly aggressive management protocols including intensive antimicrobial administrations and the provision of a well-balanced nutritional, higher caloric diet [20, 21]. The cooccurrence of tuberculosis adds another complication related to the decrease in the sensitivity of tuberculin skin test (TST), which is used as an indicator for management. This issue is aggravated further in immune-compromised children from HIV and severe malnutrition; there is a block of the immune reaction, type IV hypersensitivity, needed for a reactive TST, consequently affecting the appropriate management protocol [20, 21].

In addition, it was documented that the energy needs increase in HIV-infected children compared to normal children by almost 10% in the early stage of the disease. However, such an increased demand will go up to 20–30% in symptomatic HIV with opportunistic infections and to 50–100% in case of severe malnutrition. These data are based on studies in HIV-infected adults or in non-HIV-infected children and, therefore, have a low level of evidence [2]. A major finding of these studies is that HIV-infected children with SAM present with significant reductions in the adipocytokines, leptin, and adiponectin that are associated with mortality during inpatient hospitalization. In addition, HIV-infected and HIV-negative patients presented with similar degrees of wasting and edema, who achieved similar rates of growth and recovery [22]. Accordingly, as evidenced in **Table 1**, a baseline metabolic profile including amino acid levels was suggested for HIV-infected and HIV-negative patients [22].

5. Nutrition as an adjunct therapy

The introduction of therapeutic nutrition support and appropriate fluid rehydration has improved the rehabilitation process, shortened hospital stays of HIV-uninfected severely malnourished children, and addressed micronutrient and macronutrient deficiencies [19]. In the stabilization phase, F-75 is given as a therapeutic food. It is a low-protein milk-based formula diet. It is followed gradually by F-100 over a couple of days. The transitional phase until rehabilitation phase is reached. F-100 is a milk formula with higher protein and energy content than F75. However, the ready-to-use therapeutic food (RUTF) has replaced the F-100, especially in cases of severe acute malnutrition. In general, RUTF are pastes, no liquids, containing a combination of milk powder, electrolytes, and micronutrients. They provide the child with the same nutrients as F-100 plus iron [3, 4, 7]. As for rehydration, ReSoMal is commonly used. It contains approximately 45 mmol Na, 40 mmol K, and 3 mmol Mg per liter [19]. However, the metabolic and nutrient needs of HIV-infected children, in whom persistent anorexia is frequent, should be more clearly defined. In case of severe diarrhea often associated with high mortality rates, the provision of suitable feeding protocols is highly recommended. In brief, protocols for appropriate nutrition support therapy for severely malnourished infants below age 6 months are needed [23].

Although wasting can be treated in HIV-uninfected children with nutritional therapy alone, effective regimens for HIV-infected children need to be developed.

The use of high-energy therapeutic nutrition support (e.g., F100 or RUTF) is part of standard care that can start the soonest regardless of the ART starting date. However, high mortality (38%), within 4–6 weeks, remains an issue. Many children will gain weight with nutrition support alone. Sometimes, CD4 cell count could be used to monitor the nutritional needs and to identify those needing treatment [15]. However, other reports pointed out that CD4 cell counts do not seem to improve after the provision of nutritional therapy. In brief, community therapeutic care methods, strengthened by local production of ready-to-use therapeutic foods, require fewer staff to run programs and ensure compliance. It is also worth noting that the HIV epidemic has generated a new group of children requiring nutrition rehabilitation unit-based care [20].

The situation becomes more complicated when opportunistic infections enter the picture, necessitating the use of anti-infective medications in malnourished children. Such drugs have a wide range of toxicity, which worsen the nutritional status of the children [18, 21]. Such children require urgent stabilization of multiple physiological parameters including hypoglycemia, dehydration, and electrolyte imbalance. Nutritional support is generally tailored to each case with consideration given to the rate of weight gain [10, 21].

Although interventions with multiple nutritional regimens increase energy and protein intake, in such situations, they led to no improvement in the morbidity and mortality rates compared to placebo. Observational studies have reported that the recovery from acute malnutrition and underweight using ready-to-use therapeutic food (RUTF) in populations of malnourished children, including some infected with HIV, was often complete with these products [2, 17, 19]. It was also noted that severe wasting makes the clinical assessment of dehydration difficult, so the presence of metabolic acidosis and lethargy are often the clinical indications available to prompt rehydration and nutritional interventions. Unfortunately, there are also currently inadequate data on the optimum regimen of supportive care (e.g., for shock) in the malnourished child who has adapted to a reduced body mass and organ system function. Appropriate dietary therapies are needed for this increasing population, as the standard F-75 and F-100 formulas are likely unsuitable [3, 21]; they might lead to the refeeding syndrome. Refeeding syndrome can be defined as the potentially fatal shifts in fluids and electrolytes that may occur in malnourished patients receiving artificial refeeding whether enterally or parenterally [19].

Besides, in Jesson and Leroy review, vitamin A was used as a primary therapy; it decreased pediatric mortality by 50% whatever the cause and improved short-term growth, in untreated HIV-infected children in Tanzania [2].

6. Antiretroviral therapy (ART) and nutrition

It is well documented that the availability of highly active antiviral therapy (HAART) for the past two decades or so has decreased remarkably the mortality and morbidity of the disease in both adults and children, thus transforming it into a chronic infections disease [9]. The prognosis of HIV-infected children has markedly improved in the HAART era, both in terms of morbidity and mortality as mentioned earlier, despite the fact the mortality rate in HIV-infected children is still considerably higher than the pediatric general population [9, 23].

In Tanzania, when ART became available, the recovery was improved, especially when ART was initiated in children at the same time as nutritional support than when it was initiated later [2].

In the literature, there seems to be conflicting recommendations about when and how to begin nutrition support with ART. Some studies have reported that if ART is started when children have severe wasting due to malnutrition, they have higher rates of mortality compared to those with less clinical markers of malnutrition. However, studies were not conclusive about the time to start nutritional support [5, 15]. A recent retrospective study finding suggests that starting ART early in malnourished children results in higher rates of nutritional recovery and weight gain than if ART is delayed. In a study performed on a cohort of children in Africa, 59% of Zambian children were initially underweight and almost three quarters (72%) had slowed down or stopped growth when ART was administered. In these children, prominent improvements in both weight and height were recorded when nutritional support started in the initial stage after diagnosis at the same time as ART. In fact, the best increase was observed among children who were most underweight. Therefore, these lifesaving medications should not be delayed, and child health systems should embrace this approach in a programmatic manner [5, 21].

On the other hand, ART in children has been reported to result in metabolic disorders, which negatively affect the nutrition status, particularly, at the initiation and first few months of treatment. Such side effects include nausea, vomiting, dysregulated lipid metabolism [5, 11], low bond density, and increased fractures [11, 22]. Consequently, at the initiation of ART, the nutritional status must be evaluated, particularly that about half of the children taking such treatment will be underweight. Such a condition could lead to chronic malnutrition of about two-thirds of HIV-infected children in countries with limited resources with a higher two to three times risk of death.

Nutritional evaluation, monitoring, and support are strongly recommended, especially at the initiation period and the first 2 months. Such measures proved to decrease morbidity and mortality [2, 10]. Children severely immunodeficient at initiation of ART may have a better growth outcome than nonimmunodeficient children at initiation. Children treated with ART become less immunodeficient, and their nutritional status improves [2]. In general, protease inhibitors (PI)-based treatments result in decreasing viral load, less resistant mutation, and better growth compared to non-PI-based regimens. Many authors focusing on this issue have reported that the earlier the treatment was initiated in children, the better the nutritional response in weight and height was [2, 23]. Malnourished children treated with ART may develop a kwashiorkor-like syndrome of IRIS (immune reconstitution inflammatory syndrome) [21]. However, in children with severe malnutrition, there has been a concern that standard dosing of ART may be inappropriate. This concern is based on the malnourishment metabolic alterations that could lead to subtherapeutic or toxic drug levels that may contribute to viral resistance and/or safety issues [2, 5, 14].

Implementation challenges in starting and maintaining children on ART also persist and are found throughout the chain of care in sub-Saharan Africa, especially in rural areas [21].

7. Recommendations

In children, transmission of HIV through breastfeeding remains a problem. Efforts have moved in support of safer feeding by promoting exclusive breastfeeding for 6 months coupled with concomitant antiretroviral prophylaxis delivered to breastfeeding mothers or the infant [1, 18]. However, nutritional management of HIV-infected children remains a challenge in view of all the studies reviewed.

HIV-positive women living in resource-poor environments must balance opposing risks. In 2010, the WHO revised its position by recommending exclusive breastfeeding for the first 6 months of life followed by complementary foods and then accompanied by postnatal infant or maternal antiretroviral prophylaxis (WHO). In contrast, the American Academy of Pediatrics recommends that HIV-infected mothers not to breastfeed their infants, regardless of maternal disease status, viral load, or ART and the British HIV association concurs [1, 18].

The important issue is to meet all nutrient needs and provide the required energy requirements. However, according to the WHO, some considerations are needed for safely replacing food. Such considerations are based on the fact that untreated HIV-infected patients have an increased resting energy expenditure, decreased appetite, digestion of food, and absorption of nutrients. In brief, such patients often have a range of micronutrient deficiencies. However, there are no evidence-based guidelines on the appropriate types and amounts of micronutrient supplements for HIV-infected children. The WHO has previously endorsed the use of ready-to-use therapeutic foods to reduce mortality and undernutrition [18].

8. Conclusion

In the area of nutrition and HIV, children deserve special attention because of their additional needs to ensure growth and development and their dependency on adults for adequate care. Nutritional advice and support should be a priority component of the continuum of care for HIV-infected women and children. Furthermore, case by case, the special nutritional needs of children should be determined in light of the guidelines and recommendations adopted by various professional health and medical associations. Wasting and undernutrition in HIV-infected children reflect a series of failures within the health system, the home, and the community and not just a biological process related to virus and host interactions. In brief, despite the great impact of recent pharmacologic interventions, optimal nutrition continues to be essential therapy for HIV-infected children, and it has the potential to provide adjunct immune-modulatory therapy, thus improving care and outcomes of children with HIV/AIDS.

Author details

Inaya Hajj Hussein[1*], Lara Youssef[2], Andrea Mladenovic[3], Angelo Leone[4], Abdo Jurjus[5] and Virginia Uhley[1]

1 Department of Foundational Medical Studies, Oakland University William Beaumont School of Medicine, Rochester, MI, USA

2 Faculty of Nursing and Health Sciences, Notre Dame University, Lebanon

3 School of Medicine, University of Belgrade, Belgrade, Serbia

4 Department of Experimental and Clinical Neurosciences, University of Palermo, Palermo, Italy

5 Department of Anatomy, Cell Biology and Physiological Sciences, Faculty of Medicine, American University of Beirut, Beirut, Lebanon

*Address all correspondence to: hajjhuss@oakland.edu

IntechOpen

References

[1] Saloojee H, Cooper P. HIV and AIDS. World Review of Nutrition and Dietetics. 2015;**113**:173-177. DOI: 10.1159/000360332

[2] Jesson J, Leroy V. Challenges of malnutrition care among HIV-infected children on antiretroviral treatment in Africa. Médecine et Maladies Infectieuses. 2015;**45**(5):149-156. DOI: 10.1016/j.medmal.2015.03.002

[3] Butensky EA. The role of nutrition in pediatric HIV/AIDS: A review of micronutrient research. Journal of Pediatric Nursing. 2001;**16**(6):402-411. DOI: 10.1053/jpdn.2001.27881

[4] Deatrick JA, Lipman TH, Thurber F, Ash L, Carlino H, McKnight H, et al. Nutritional assessment for children who are HIV-infected. Pediatric Nursing. 1998;**24**(2):137-141, 149

[5] Ebissa G, Deyessa N, Biadgilign S. Impact of highly active antiretroviral therapy on nutritional and immunologic status in HIV-infected children in the low-income country of Ethiopia. Nutrition. 2016;**32**(6):667-673. DOI: 10.1016/j.nut.2015.12.035

[6] Global HIV & AIDS statistics—2018 fact sheet. 2019. UNAIDS. Available from: http://www.unaids.org/en/resources/fact-sheet

[7] Spira R, Lepage P, Msellati P, Van De Perre P, Leroy V, Simonon A, et al. Natural history of human immunodeficiency virus type 1 infection in children: A five-year prospective study in Rwanda. Mother-to-child HIV-1 transmission study group. Pediatrics. 1999;**104**(5):e56

[8] Newell ML, Coovadia H, Cortina-Borja M, Rollins N, Gaillard P, Dabis F; Ghent International AIDS Society (IAS) Working Group on HIV Infection in Women and Children Mortality of infected and uninfected infants born to HIV-infected mothers in Africa: A pooled analysis. Lancet. 2004;**364**(9441):1236-1243

[9] Berti E, Thorne C, Noguera-Julian A, Rojo P, Galli L, de Martino M, et al. The new face of the pediatric HIV epidemic in Western countries: Demographic characteristics, morbidity and mortality of the pediatric HIV-infected population. The Pediatric Infectious Disease Journal. 2015;**34**(5 Suppl 1):S7-S13. DOI: 10.1097/INF.0000000000000660

[10] Clark WA, Cress EM. Nutritional issues and positive living in human immunodeficiency virus/AIDS. The Nursing Clinics of North America. 2018;**53**(1):13-24. DOI: 10.1016/j.cnur.2017.10.002

[11] Penazzato M, Prendergast AJ, Muhe LM, Tindyebwa D, Abrams E. Optimisation of antiretroviral therapy in HIV-infected children under 3 years of age. Cochrane Database of Systematic Reviews. 2014;**5**:CD004772. DOI: 10.1002/14651858.CD004772.pub4

[12] Fenner L, Brinkhof MW, Keiser O, Weigel R, Cornell M, Moultrie H, et al. International epidemiologic databases to evaluate AIDS in Southern Africa. Early mortality and loss to follow-up in HIV-infected children starting antiretroviral therapy in southern Africa. Journal of Acquired Immune Deficiency Syndromes. 2010;**54**(5):524-532. DOI: 10.1097/QAI.0b013e3181e0c4cf

[13] Davies MA, May M, Bolton-Moore C, et al. Prognosis of children with HIV-1 infection starting antiretroviral therapy in southern Africa: A collaborative analysis of treatment programs. The Pediatric Infectious Disease Journal. 2014;**33**:608. DOI: 10.1097/INF.0000000000000214

[14] Nnyepi M, Bennink MR, Jackson-Malete J, Sumathi Venkatesh S, Malete L, Mokgatlhe L, et al. Nutrition status of HIV+ children in Botswana. Health Education. 2015;**115**(5):495-514. DOI: 10.1108/HE-04-2014-0052

[15] Duggal S, Chugh TD, Duggal AK. HIV and malnutrition: Effects on immune system. Clinical & Developmental Immunology. 2012;**2012**:784740. DOI: 10.1155/2012/784740

[16] Okechukwu A, Okechukwu O, Chiaha I. Burden of HIV infection in children with severe acute malnutrition at the University of Abuja Teaching Hospital Gwagwalada, Nigeria. Journal of HIV for Clinical and Scientific Research. 2015;**2**(3):055-061. DOI: 10.17352/2455-3786.000015

[17] Saunders J, Smith T, Stroud M. Malnutrition and undernutrition. Medicine. 2015;**43**(2):112-118

[18] United Nations Children's Fund, World Health Organization, World Bank. UNICEF-WHO-World Bank Joint Child Malnutrition Estimates. New York, USA/Geneva, Switzerland/Washington DC, USA: UNICEF/WHO/World Bank; 2012

[19] Friis H, Michaelsen KF. Micronutrients and HIV infection: A review. European Journal of Clinical Nutrition. 1998;**52**(3):157-163

[20] Heikens GT, Bunn J, Amadi B, Manary M, Chhagan M, Berkley JA, et al. Case management of HIV-infected severely malnourished children: Challenges in the area of highest prevalence. Lancet. 2008;**371**(9620):1305-1307. DOI: 10.1016/S0140-6736(08)60565-6

[21] Trehan I, O'Hare BA, Phiri A, Heikens GT. Challenges in the management of HIV-infected malnourished children in sub-Saharan Africa. AIDS Research and Treatment. 2012;**2012**:790786. DOI: 10.1155/2012/790786

[22] Mody A, Bartz S, Hornik CP, Kiyimba T, Bain J, Muehlbauer M, et al. Effects of HIV infection on the metabolic and hormonal status of children with severe acute malnutrition. PLoS One. 2014;**9**(7):e102233. DOI: 10.1371/journal.pone.0102233

[23] Saghayam S, Wanke C. The impact of nutritional status and nutrition supplementation on outcomes along the HIV treatment cascade in the resource-limited setting. Current Opinion in HIV and AIDS. 2015;**10**(6):472-476. DOI: 10.1097/COH.0000000000000202

Chapter 3

Malnutrition in HIV/AIDS: Aetiopathogenesis

Vangal K. Sashindran and Rajneesh Thakur

Abstract

HIV/AIDS can cause malnutrition directly and also indirectly through opportunistic infections (OIs). Infectious diarrhoea and tuberculosis are the commonest
OIs linked to malnutrition in HIV/AIDS. Environmental enteric dysfunction has
now been identified to play a significant role in HIV-malnutrition. Food insecurity
is bidirectionally associated with aggravation and perpetuation of HIV infection.
Increasingly, drugs used in antiretroviral therapy have been recognised to lead
malnutrition in many ways. Both HIV and malnutrition are most prevalent in
the poorest areas of the world, and there is a convergence of etiological factors.
Malnutrition depresses every aspect of immune function. Deficiency of key micronutrients like iron, folic acid, zinc, selenium and vitamins A, C and D also adversely
affects immune function. Recent research has led to a greater understanding of
these mechanisms. Immune dysfunction secondary to malnutrition is referred to as
nutrition-associated immunodeficiency. Hence it is easy to surmise that malnutrition and HIV/AIDs are a deadly duo.

Keywords: HIV/AIDS, malnutrition, immunity, environmental enteric dysfunction

1. Introduction

HIV/AIDS and malnutrition form a deadly duo with each one fuelling the other.
Malnutrition increases susceptibility to infection by causing immune dysfunction
in manifold ways. The depressed immune status can amplify HIV replication and
accelerate progression of HIV disease to AIDS. Malnutrition increases the risk of
death on initiation of ART in PLHA, and untreated HIV/AIDS puts individuals at
risk for malnutrition. The same is more acute in infants and children under 5 years
of age [1, 2]. Untreated or advanced HIV/AIDS is again associated with a compromised immune status that makes these patients susceptible to opportunistic infections. Of these, tuberculosis is the most common and most debilitating one. Apart
from TB, common infections like pneumonia, kala-azar, meningitis and malaria are
also more common in these patients. Infections and the chronic low-grade inflammatory state perpetuated by HIV infection suppress appetite, increase catabolism
of muscles and push patients towards malnutrition. Loss of strength means low
earning capacity and loss of livelihood. The social stigma of HIV fractures social
and family bonds. All of them further push patients towards impoverishment and
malnutrition.

2. Magnitude of the problem

A study in 2010 estimated that more than 925 million people in the world were undernourished and one-third of the global disease burden could be eliminated by adequate nutrition [3]. The greatest burden of malnutrition is seen in the age group of 2–5 years. According to 2014 data, 159 million children were stunted and 50 million were wasted [4]. Among different geographic regions, South Asia and sub-Saharan Africa have the highest global burden of malnutrition. In 2014, they accounted for 25.1 and 32% of stunted children under 5 years of age, respectively [5, 6]. Sub-Saharan Africa suffers from a high burden of undernutrition, affecting 23.2% of its population, and in 2015 this region accounted for 69% of the estimated people living with HIV globally. A review of case records of 4350 children aged 2 – 19 years enrolled in HIV-care programme in Benin, Burundi, Cameroon, Chad, Cote d'Ivoire, Mali and Togo was done in 2011. The mean age was 10 years (IQR 7 – 13). Anthropometric indices that were measured were height-for-age z-score (HAZ) and weight-for-height z-score (WHZ) for children < 5 years and BMI-for-age z-score (BAZ) for children >5 years. All values were expressed as z-scores. About 80% of the children were on ART for a median period of 36 months. The prevalence of malnutrition was 42% (95% CI 40–44%). About half of all children in the age group of 2–5 were malnourished, and among children in the age groups of 5–10 and 10–19, the prevalence was 36 and 44%, respectively. The authors then subtyped malnutrition as acute, chronic or mixed. Acute malnutrition was defined as WHZ/BAZ < −2SD and HAZ ≥ −2SD. The prevalence of acute, chronic and mixed malnutrition was 9 (95% CI 6–12%), 26 (95% CI 23–28%) and 7% (95% CI 5–10%), respectively. Acute malnutrition was associated with age < 5 years, male sex, severe immunodeficiency and absence of ART. Chronic malnutrition was most common in children <5 years (37%). The prevalence of chronic malnutrition in the age groups 5–10 and 10-19 years was 24% each. Mixed malnutrition was associated with male sex, age < 5 years, severe immunodeficiency and recent initiation of ART (<6 m) [7]. In another study from Ethiopia, malnutrition was seen in 224 of the 372 children with HIV/AIDS (60.2%). Of all the malnourished children, 67.7% were males and 52.7% were females. In the age group of 2–5 years, 96.3% were malnourished, and in the age groups of 5–10 and 10–15 years, it was 48.3 and 59.2%, respectively [8].

In a study from North India, 56.7% of 102 HIV-positive children presenting to an ART clinic had protein-energy malnutrition (PEM). Children with higher grades of PEM had lower CD4 cell counts [9]. Of the 4105 children initiating ART in TREAT Asia Paediatric HIV Observational Database (TApHOD) cohort, 355 (11.9%) had severe malnutrition (defined as baseline weight-for-height z-score of <−3 if aged 6–60 months or BMI-for-age z-score of <−3 if aged 61 months to 14 years) [10]. This is very high compared with the estimated prevalence of severe malnutrition in the general paediatric population in SE Asia (5.2%) [11]. The risk factors for severe malnutrition were age 6–12 months, male sex and prior diagnosis of tuberculosis [10].

Among adult patients, moderate malnutrition is more common than severe malnutrition. A study done in Salvador, Brazil, looked at prevalence of malnutrition in PLHA in the age group of 20–59 years. One hundred twenty-seven patients were enrolled in the study. Malnutrition (BMI < 18.5 kg/m^2) was found in 55 (43%) of the subjects and severe malnutrition (BMI < 16 kg/m^2) in 15%. Lean body mass and fat body mass were lower than the fifth percentile of a reference population in 80 (63%) and 38 (30%) patients, respectively [12]. Another study from Iran compared malnutrition among adults with HIV/AIDS with the general population. One hundred PLHA were enrolled in the study. Mild (BMI 17–18.4 kg/m^2), moderate (BMI

16–6.9 kg/m^2) and severe malnutrition (BMI < 16 kg/m^2) were seen in 24, 38 and 15%, respectively. Except for mild malnutrition, all the other figures were significantly higher than that for the general population [13]. Data from the Nutrition for Healthy Living (NFHL) cohort in Boston, USA, reveals some disturbing facts about HIV-malnutrition in the era of HAART. The total prevalence of HIV-associated weight loss and wasting in the cohort was 38%. Both weight loss and wasting were seen in those who were on a robust ART regimen, those who had failed ART and those who were ART-naive. The authors also found that the prevalence of weight loss and wasting had not changed over time and that it was as frequent in 2005 as it had been in 1997 [14].

3. Impact of HIV-malnutrition: mortality and morbidity

Malnutrition contributes to increased mortality among children, mainly due to infections. Children with severe acute malnutrition had 12 times the risk of dying when compared with well-nourished children of the same age [15]. HIV infection further increases the risk of dying among children with malnutrition. A systematic review and meta-analysis of 17 studies on 4891 children with severe acute malnutrition in sub-Saharan Africa revealed that children with HIV infection were more likely to die than those not infected with HIV (30.4 vs. 8.4%, P < 0.001, relative risk 2.81, 95% CI 2.04–3.87) [16]. Non-immunological factors also contribute to increased mortality among children with malnutrition. These include impaired respiratory excursions due to reduced muscle mass predisposing to chest infections, reduced electrolyte absorption from the gut, impaired renal concentration capacity which puts the child at risk for dehydration and lastly impaired cardiac function that can cause heart failure [17]. The NHFL study showed that for every 1% increase in weight loss since the previous visit, the risk of death rose by 11%. When weight loss was >10% below the baseline weight, the relative risk of death increased nearly sixfold [14].

4. Aetiopathogenesis of HIV-malnutrition

4.1 HIV infection per se and HIV wasting syndrome

HIV wasting was included as an AIDS-defining criterion (ADC) in 1987 by the Centers for Disease Control and Prevention (CDC). HIV wasting is defined as an involuntary weight loss of >10% from the baseline and associated with diarrhoea, fever or weakness of ≥30 days duration in the absence of a concurrent illness. HIV wasting is associated with disease progression and death even when patient is on effective ART [18]. Wasting is associated with low serum albumin levels and deficiency of important micronutrients like zinc and selenium [13].

The primary cause for weight loss in PLHA is inadequate calorie intake. One of the key factors leading to this is anorexia secondary to elevated levels of pro-inflammatory cytokines like interleukin-1 (IL-1), interleukin-6 (IL-6) and tumour necrosis factor-α (TNF-α). These cytokines also cause a rise in total daily energy expenditure (TEE) due to an increase in resting metabolic rate (RMR) or resting energy expenditure (REE) [19, 20]. RMR may increase by 10–30%, more so in the presence of concurrent infections or high viraemia and increased catabolism of proteins [14, 21–25]. Macallan et al. evaluated patients with HIV/AIDS for TEE, REE and energy intake. The REE was 9.6% higher in HIV-infected men than in HIV-negative men (25.0 vs. 22.8 kcal/kg/d; p = 0.002). But the mean TEE in HIV-infected men was lower than that of the population standard for HIV-negative men between

30 and 39 years of age (2750 kcal/d versus 3420 kcal/d) The authors concluded that this was due to reduced physical activity. However, there is a net negative energy balance because reduced TEE does not offset decreased energy intake due to anorexia and malabsorption [19]. Roubenoff and colleagues showed that cytokines released from activated PBMCs like TNF-α and IL-1β independently predicted loss of lean body mass and changes in REE [26]. And, nutritional and metabolic abnormalities correlated better with cytokines from PBMCs than plasma cytokines. Levels of TNF-α and IL-1β and IL-6 from PBMCs were better than plasma cytokines in distinguishing between participants with or without HIV wasting [27].

4.2 Anorexia

Various causes of anorexia leading to HIV wasting include oral candidiasis, oesophageal candidiasis, CMV oesophagitis, fever and tuberculosis. ART is also associated with significant adverse effects that include anorexia. Many NRTIs cause mitochondrial toxicity. Lactic acidosis and pancreatitis are two of the most serious effects of mitochondrial toxicity due to NRTIs, especially didanosine, stavudine and zidovudine. Frank lactic acidosis is not common, but hyperlacticacidaemia is fairly common and is seen in about 15% of patients on these NRTIs. It manifests with anorexia, nausea, weight loss, peripheral lipoatrophy and mildly deranged transaminitis. Zidovudine causes anorexia, nausea and fatigue in 5–10% patients during the early stages of therapy. Other drugs associated with anorexia and nausea include ritonavir and elvitegravir-cobicistat combination [28, 29]. Anorexia may also be secondary to jaundice secondary to HBV/HCV coinfection. Many ART drugs can cause hepatitis by different mechanisms. NRTIs cause steatohepatitis by mitochondrial toxicity. This usually develops after 6 months of treatment. NNRTIs cause hepatitis by hypersensitivity reaction. This usually occurs within the first 2–4 months of therapy. Protease inhibitors may cause hepatitis especially with HBV or HCV confection by an unknown mechanism. Anti-tubercular therapy is also another significant cause of iatrogenic hepatitis. Alcoholism, drug abuse and depression may all be associated with anorexia.

4.3 Chronic diarrhoea

Diarrhoea remains a common complaint among PLHA and adversely affects quality of life. In the early years of the HIV epidemic, HIV wasting syndrome was a common presentation, especially in sub-Saharan Africa. It would often be associated with prolonged diarrhoea (>30 days duration). Causes for diarrhoea can be infectious and non-infectious. In most of the low-income countries, the aetiology continues to be infectious, and etiologic agents differ according to geographical region [30, 31]. The aetiological agents can be broadly grouped as protozoa, bacteria, fungi and viruses.

4.3.1 Infectious diarrhoea

Cryptosporidium parvum is the most frequently identified protozoan causing chronic diarrhoea in PLHA universally [32]. In developing countries, prevalence rates of cryptosporidium infection can be as high as 20% [33]. The high prevalence is due to sewage/faecal contamination of water sources [34]. Although cryptosporidium is commonly associated with chronic diarrhoea in HIV-positive persons, it can also cause cholera-like explosive diarrhoea and intermittent acute and relapsing illnesses. Microsporidia (*Enterocytozoon bieneusi* and *Encephalitozoon intestinalis*) are other important protozoa causing diarrhoea in AIDS patients [35–38]. In a study from New York, microsporidia were found in 39% of AIDS patients undergoing gastrointestinal evaluation for diarrhoea [39]. But this high prevalence is uncommon in other parts of the USA and the rest of the world [36]. *Isospora belli* is an endemic gastrointestinal pathogen among PLHA in Haiti, but it is uncommon in the USA [36, 37]. The widespread use of trimethoprim-co-trimoxazole prophylaxis for *Pneumocystis carinii* may be the reason for this low prevalence: *Isospora* being very susceptible to trimethoprim-sulphamethoxazole. Cyclospora have also been identified in HIV-infected patients with chronic diarrhoea in low- to middle-income countries (LMIC) [35–37]. Amoebic dysentery or invasive amoebic disease like liver abscess or amoeboma is not more common in PLHA than in the general population even in developing countries. A high frequency of stool carriage in asymptomatic homosexual men is however common [30]. Stool carriage of amoebae in PLHA includes *E. dispar*, *E. hartmanni*, *E. coli* and also non-pathogenic *E. histolytica* [40]. There is no difference in the prevalence or severity of giardiasis among PLHA and HIV-negative populations.

The spectrum of bacterial pathogens causing diarrhoea in HIV-infected patients is similar to that in the general population. *Salmonella*, *Shigella*, *Campylobacter* and *E. coli* remain the commonest causes of diarrhoea in PLHA also. The immunocompromised state can lead to a symptomatic carriage of *Shigella* and *Campylobacter* [30]. *Clostridium difficile* should be actively excluded in patients with recent history of antibiotic therapy [41]. Clostridial infection is more common in severely immunocompromised patients (CD4+ T-cell count <50/ mm^3). *Mycobacterium avium* complex (MAC) typically causes diarrhoea in patients with AIDS with profound immunosuppression (i.e. CD4+ T-cell count <50 cells/mm^3) [42]. Features of systemic involvement in the form of fever and weight loss often accompany diarrhoea [43]. MAC usually involves the small intestine; however, it can affect the entire GI tract [44, 45].

Fungi are rare etiologic agents for diarrhoea in HIV-infected. The only exception is histoplasmosis which can infect all parts of the GIT; can cause fever, weight loss and diarrhoea; and may require hospitalisation [46].

Cytomegalovirus (CMV) was identified in as many as 45% of GI biopsies in AIDS patients with diarrhoea in a study from France [47]. CMV infection usually presents late in the natural history of HIV/AIDS, occurring when CD4 count is <100 cells/mm^3. In contrast, CMV was not detected in any of the rectal biopsies from 29 African patients with chronic diarrhoea and abnormally appearing rectal mucosa [48]. Other viruses that have been identified in stools of PLHA with chronic diarrhoea include adenovirus, rotavirus, astrovirus, picornavirus and coronavirus [49, 50]. An Italian study followed up a cohort of 50 HIV-negative and 10 HIV-positive children for 1 year and collected stool samples from the children every alternate week. The samples were tested for rotavirus (RV), and they found that while HIV-positive children shed more RV in stools, these rotaviral infections were not more often associated with diarrhoea than in HIV-negative children [51]. Similar prevalence was also reported from Lusaka in Zambia and Baltimore in the USA [52, 53].

Chronic *Strongyloides* infection may be present as chronic diarrhoea. *Strongyloides* hyper-infection can occur in the immunocompromised. Disseminated *Strongyloides* infection leads to migration of larvae into various tissues outside the gut. The migrating larvae carry gut bacteria along, leading to bacterial translocation which can trigger systemic inflammation and sepsis [54].

4.3.2 Non-infectious diarrhoea

4.3.2.1 ART-induced diarrhoea

With early diagnosis and institution of antiretroviral therapy, the incidence of infective diarrhoea has declined, and non-infectious causes are being increasingly identified. The common causes now are ART-associated diarrhoea, HIV enteropathy and causes seen in the general population. About 60% of patients receiving ART gave history of diarrhoea in the previous month [55]. Data from clinical trials suggest that up to 19% of these events may have been due to the adverse effects of ART [56]. Among the ART drugs, protease inhibitors (PIs) seem to be most strongly associated with diarrhoea. In mouse models, PIs and reverse transcriptase inhibitors significantly increased water and electrolyte secretion into intestinal lumen *in vivo* [57]. Rufo and colleagues demonstrated that protease inhibitors in general, and nelfinavir in particular, potentiate signalling through muscarinic and calcium-dependent receptors of intestinal cells leading to increased chloride secretion into the lumen [58]. Stool samples of these patients also had increased concentrations of sodium and chloride consistent with secretory diarrhoea. In an *in vitro* study, Bode and colleagues showed that PIs induced apoptosis of human intestinal epithelium, thereby compromising barrier function and increasing water secretion in gut lumen. Decreased alkaline phosphatase activity in cells exposed to PIs led to accumulation of unfolded proteins in the cytosol. A failure of the cell's 'unfolded protein response', a specific signalling pathway aimed at returning the cell's protein folding function back to normal, triggered cellular apoptosis [59]. Wu and colleagues found that lopinavir and ritonavir induced endoplasmic reticulum dysfunction in intestinal epithelial cells that led to diarrhoea [60].

4.3.2.2 HIV enteropathy

HIV enteropathy is an idiopathic form of diarrhoea observed in all stages of HIV disease in the absence of an infectious source and with characteristic histologic features [61–63]. Changes include crypt epithelial proliferation leading to increased crypt height, later crypt cell encroachment onto villi and relative decreased villous height. The consequence of these changes are diarrhoea and malabsorption [64, 65]. While the exact mechanisms by which these changes occur in the GI tract are unclear, HIV has been postulated to alter signalling and cellular structure, which may lead to architectural distortion [61]. Keating and colleagues investigated monosaccharide absorption in patients with HIV and AIDS. They demonstrated that patients with diarrhoea had significant malabsorption of all monosaccharides tested [66]. Malabsorption occurred irrespective of pathogen-positive or pathogen-negative diarrhoea, indicating that HIV had an independent direct role. This may be due to the ability of HIV to infect mucosal epithelial cells [67]. Increased mucosal infiltration by activated CD8+ T cells results in high levels of pro-inflammatory cytokines which can directly damage the mucosal barrier [61, 63]. Other hypotheses for the mechanism of HIV enteropathy include decreased transepithelial electrical resistance, decreased sodium-dependent glucose absorption and increased intercellular permeability in HIV-infected cells [68]. HIV enteropathy can also lead to malabsorption of vitamin B_{12}, bile acid and monosaccharides [61, 64, 68].

4.4 Environmental enteric dysfunction

Chronic diarrhoea, water, sanitation and hygiene (WASH) have been implicated as causative factors for severe stunting in low- and middle-income countries for a long time. Efficacy of WASH interventions in reducing diarrhoea and malnutrition has been lower than expected. This led to the search for another cause. Today, there is sufficient evidence that the cause is environmental enteric dysfunction (EED). It is 'an apparently seasonal and reversible disorder characterised by gut mucosal cell villous atrophy, crypt hyperplasia, increased permeability and increased inflammatory cell infiltrate'. The principal driver of EED is the high burden of intestinal infectious disease which is not enough to cause diarrhoea but enough to induce a state of chronic immune activation in the gut mucosa, thereby leading to epithelial damage. Dysbiosis of gut microbiota is also now considered to have an important role. The pathogenesis is probably chronic exposure to pathogens leading to a T cell-mediated immune response in the gut which continues to remain in an inflammatory hyperimmune state. This exaggerated immune response leads to structural changes in the gut mucosa, increased inflammation and permeability of the intestines, resulting in disrupted gut immune response; reduced absorption, delivery and utilisation of nutrients; and finally nutritional deficiency. There are also features of systemic inflammation, microbial translocation (MT) across the permeable gut mucosa and changes in the gut microbiome. Malnutrition further impairs the renewal of gut mucosal cells, maturation and proliferation of intestinal cells and pancreatic islet cells. The chronic low-grade inflammation inhibits endochondral ossification, thus inhibiting bone growth and leads to stunting [69].

The pathological hallmark of EED is villus blunting, which means that in histological sections villus height is reduced and villus width increased. Increased intestinal permeability can be detected using disaccharide probes. This is considered a diagnostic hallmark of EED. In adults confocal laser endomicroscopy (CLE) can be used to detect leakage of fluorescein dye from systemic circulation into the gut lumen. In adults with EED, CLE shows extensive leakage into the gut lumen occurring especially at the villous tips. This suggests that micro-erosions secondary to disordered epithelial cell shedding may be an important cause for the increased permeability [70]. The increased permeability leads to malabsorption of nutrients and also microbial translocation (MT) from the lumen into systemic circulation via gut mucosa. This MT is also important in perpetuating a chronic inflammatory state. Due to MT, some important biomarkers of MT are now being used to detect EED. These include bacterial cell wall lipopolysaccharide (LPS), soluble lipopolysaccharide co-receptor (sCD14) and antibodies to the LPS core antigen (EndoCAb) [71]. The clinical impact of EE, apart from stunting, is decreased immunological response to oral vaccines.

Does EED fuel HIV replication and disease progression? It is attractive to think it does so. Aggregation of intraepithelial lymphocytes and lamina propria T-cell populations has been described in children with EED. The T cells expressed CD69 and HLA-DR. Children with EED had 4–5 times more CD3+ T cells and 15–30-fold higher number of CD25+ T cells in the lamina propria than the UK controls. They also had a higher proportion of T cells than TCRαδ+ [72]. Activated lymphocytes in a milieu rich in inflammatory cytokines would be the perfect ground for HIV attachment and replication. However there have been no studies to prove or disprove this. But Jacob and his colleagues have demonstrated that the dominant effect of HIV on enteric mucosa is to increase villous crypt depth [73]. Hence HIV and EED may work synergistically to aggravate malnutrition.

4.5 Oral ulcers

Recurrent and severe oral ulcers make eating uncomfortable and painful. Decreased food intake over a period of time can precipitate malnutrition. Oral candidiasis is the most frequent oral disease associated AIDS, with a prevalence of 70–90% [74–76]. It often occurs early in the course of the disease. With decline in immune status, its frequency and severity worsens, and it may occur along with oesophageal candidiasis. Recurrent major aphthous ulcers and herpetiform aphthous ulcers are painful and adversely affect food intake. Other conditions like Kaposi sarcoma are becoming uncommon now.

4.6 Tuberculosis

Coinfection with HIV and *Mycobacterium tuberculosis* (TB) is an extremely common problem. TB is the largest single cause of death in HIV-positive individuals, and, in areas of high prevalence, it is the most common coinfection in HIV-positive children. HIV and TB pathogens interact, resulting in an accelerated clinical course and premature death. TB infection results in secondary wasting. Indeed, weight loss is the presenting feature in almost 50% of cases of TB, and persistent anorexia is a feature in approximately one-quarter. Swaminathan, Padmapriyadarsini and colleagues studied the nutritional status of HIV-positive subjects with TB (n = 174) and HIV-positive ones without TB (n = 488). They compared their nutritional status to that of HIV-negative people of the same socioeconomic status (n = 160). They found that 50% of HIV-positive subjects with TB and one-third of HIV-positive subjects without TB had a BMI of <18.5 kg/m^2. Moreover, HIV-positive subjects both with and without TB had lower mid-arm circumference, hip circumference and waist circumference than HIV-negative individuals. HIV-positive people with TB remained underweight even after adequate treatment for TB underscoring the negative impact of TB on the nutritional status of these people and also the synergistic effect of HIV-TB confection in aggravating malnutrition [77]. Furthermore, malnutrition is a risk factor for the acquisition of primary TB infection, as well as progression to active disease [78–80]. Other infections—particularly pneumonias, which are very common in HIV-positive children—have also been found to contribute to the increased risk of malnutrition in children in several lower-income countries.

4.7 HIV endocrinopathies

Adrenal insufficiency is the commonest endocrinopathy in the HIV-infected. The mechanism of primary adrenal insufficiency in the HIV-infected is twofold: HIV adrenalitis and adrenal gland destruction secondary to tuberculosis, CMV or other opportunistic infections [81]. Sepsis may also precipitate acute adrenal insufficiency. Adrenal insufficiency can also be iatrogenic, triggered by drugs like ketoconazole and rifampicin [82]. Secondary adrenal insufficiency can be due to the direct effect of HIV on the hypothalamic-pituitary-adrenal (HPA) axis also. Cytokines like interleukin-1 (IL-1), IL-6 (in a synergistic manner) and TNF-α can suppress the HPA [83]. HIV-positive patients who develop adrenal insufficiency may present either acutely or chronically. Acute insufficiency manifests in the critically ill as Addisonian crisis characterised by profound hypotension. In our study on hypoadrenalism in the HIV-infected with current or past tuberculosis, it was found that certain clinical features occurred consistently. They included history of fatigue, lethargy, muscle weakness, low mood/irritability, significant weight loss and need to micturate frequently and findings of hypotension, both resting and postural and pale skin (under publication). The prevalence of hypoadrenalism in HIV and HIV-TB varies from 20 to 70%. This is mainly because many studies were only done on critically ill patients in the hospital. The use of standard and low-dose ACTH stimulation test also made a difference in pickup. Nevertheless, wasting in an HIV-positive patient should trigger a search for adrenal insufficiency. On the other hand, in one study it was seen that testosterone deficiency does not lead to significant wasting [26].

4.8 Co-trimoxazole prophylaxis (CPT)

Severe acute malnutrition (SAM) contributes to 1 million childhood deaths annually worldwide, and its treatment is a key strategy for reducing childhood mortality [84]. Infectious disease is thought to be the main mediator of mortality in children with SAM. Trehan and colleagues studied the efficacy of empirical antimicrobial therapy in children with severe acute malnutrition but without clinical features of infection. Two thousand seven hundred sixty-seven children in the age group of 6–59 months were randomised into three arms. One received oral amoxycillin, the other cefdinir and the last group a placebo for 7 days. Twelve-week mortality rates for the three groups were 4.8, 4.1 and 7.2%, respectively. The relative risk for death for placebo compared with amoxycillin was 1.55 (95% CI 0.7–2.24) and for placebo compared with cefdinir was 1.80 (95% CI 1.22–2.64). Differences in mortality and recovery were not statistically different between the amoxycillin and cefdinir arms [85].

Daily co-trimoxazole prophylaxis reduced all-cause mortality and hospital admissions in children with HIV/AIDS. This was despite high levels of antimicrobial resistance being identified in vitro among invasive isolates at study sites [86, 87]. Co-trimoxazole protected HIV-infected children against malaria, pneumonia and sepsis [88]. Other studies have shown its role in preventing recurrent urinary tract infections, pneumonia in children with measles and infections in children with specific immunodeficiencies [89–91]. Prendergast and colleagues reported that co-trimoxazole prophylaxis retards decline in weight and height for age in HIV-infected children, not on ART [92]. Boettiger and colleagues also found that CPT may enhance weight recovery in children with malnutrition on ART [10]. In both HIV-infected and malnourished children, the beneficial effect of antimicrobial therapy is primarily due to prevention and treatment of infections. Other collateral benefits could be reduction of inflammation which would reduce diversion of nutrients and decreased cytokine-mediated growth retardation and also reduced enteropathy and perturbations of gut flora [93].

4.9 Substance abuse and psychiatric disorders

HIV infection and chronic drug abuse both compromise nutritional status. There is a synergistic effect in HIV-positive drug users that leads to wasting and significantly impacts mortality. Illicit drug use may interfere with nutrient absorption, mute appetite and alter metabolism. Lifestyle of chronic drug users may compromise their access to food, food selection, housing, family and social support [94]. Use of injection drugs correlated with lower protein intake in the NFHL cohort study [14]. IV drug can be associated with HIV-HBV or HIV-HCV coinfections. Patients with hepatitis frequently lose weight and develop anaemia and neutropenia. As liver disease advances, anorexia, dietary intolerance and limitation of nutrient intake occur [95, 96]. AIDS-related dementia and neuropsychiatric disorders can cause malnutrition as the ability of patients to care for themselves is compromised. Many may forget to eat and others may be unable to prepare balanced meals [97].

4.10 Socioeconomic factors

4.10.1 Food insecurity

Wasting and malnutrition in HIV-positive children is not only due to the HIV disease or opportunistic infections. It is also due to breakdown of family structure and the failure of social and healthcare systems. Food insecurity is defined as a lack of access to sufficient, safe and nutritious food to meet dietary needs and maintain a healthy and active life [98]. Another way of defining it is 'insufficient quantity or quality of food, reductions of food intake, and feelings of uncertainty, anxiety, or shame over food' [99].

There is a high prevalence of food insecurity among PLHA. An American study reported that about 50% of PLHA on ART in San Francisco, Atlanta and Vancouver were food insecure [100, 101]. In the NFHL cohort from Boston, 36.1% participants were classified as 'food insecure' [14]. A study done in Senegal compared the prevalence of food insecurity among general population and PLHA in two different regions of Senegal: Dakar where the predominant source of income was nonagricultural business and Ziguinchor in Casamance province where it was agriculture. The prevalence of food insecurity among PLHA in the two regions was much higher being 84.6 and 89.5%, respectively, than in the general population (16–60%). The prevalence of severe food insecurity was 59.6 and 75.4% in Dakar and Ziguinchor, respectively [102]. Similar findings are reported from both urban and rural settings in other parts of Africa. Among 898 PLHA on ART in Kinshasa, Democratic Republic of Congo, 57% of the people were food insecure and 50.9% were severely food insecure [103]. The prevalence is higher in other studies. In one from Windhoek, Namibia, 92% of 390 PLHA on ART were food insecure, and 67% were severely food insecure [104]. In a big study involving 76,038 HIV-infected people in Western Kenya, the prevalence of food insecurity ranged from 20 to 50% [105]. The prevalence of food insecurity in rural Uganda and North Ethiopia were 74.5 and 40.4%, respectively [106, 107].

Food insecurity is linked to lower educational levels and low socioeconomic status, unemployment, larger household size and number of children [108, 109]. Andrade and colleagues found that daily per capita income correlates well with malnutrition in Salvador, Brazil. They found that for daily per capital incomes of <US$ 2, US$ 2–4.99 and US$ 5–9.99, the prevalence of malnutrition increased by 2.01 (95% CI 1.06–3.81), 1.75 (95% CI 0.92–3.35) and 1.42 (95% CI 0.76–2.65) times, respectively, compared to the patients whose *per capita* household income was US$ ≥10.00 per day [12]. The presence of even one HIV-positive person in a family pushes the family to food insecurity in Africa [110]. In most of Africa, South America and Asia, women are the primary caregivers in households. They procure foodstuffs, gather firewood, prepare food and feed the children. Not surprisingly, the risk of malnutrition in children increases if the mother has HIV/AIDS. Timely provision of ART to HIV-positive women reduces under-5 mortality rates to those similar to children of HIV-negative women.

HIV/AIDS is a major factor leading to food insecurity. The disease leads to debility of family members in the prime of their life. This leads to loss of jobs, reduced productivity and increased caregiver burden. In turn, food insecurity has many adverse effects on health and well-being of PLHA. It leads to risky coping strategies in households with HIV-positive individuals. Wages get directed to purchase of ART, and many family members may exchange sex for money or food, thereby putting themselves at higher risk of acquiring HIV infection and STDs. It also increases risk of vertical transmission of HIV by risky infant-feeding practices. It increases non-adherence to ART, aggravates adverse effects of ART, and leads to incomplete viral suppression, worsening health and increased mortality [111, 112]. In DRC and Namibia, food insecurity was associated with increased odds of poor adherence to ART (adjusted odds ratio 2.06 and odds ratio 3.84) [103, 104].

4.10.2 Poor weaning practices.

Mothers' level of education influences occurrence of malnutrition in children. Poor education leads to lack of awareness of the importance of exclusive breast feeding for the first 6 months of the infant's life, failure to introduce complementary feeds at 6 months and limited food diversity. It also contributes to adherence to local taboos with regard to refraining from giving foods of animal origin to children.

In addition, lack of access to food supplements for HIV-positive children also contributes to malnutrition among these children in many parts of Africa [113]. Exclusive breast feeding during first 6 weeks of life resulted in consistently higher z-scores for weight at 52 weeks of age in HIV-infected infants than in those on only top feeds or mixed feeds (difference of 130 g for male children and 110 g for female children) [1].

5. Pathobiology of immunodeficiency in malnutrition

Malnutrition is considered to be the commonest cause of immunodeficiency in the world. It adversely impacts every aspect of immune function. All these immune dysfunctions are collectively referred to as nutritional-acquired immunodeficiency syndrome (NAIDS). Understanding of malnutrition-related immunodeficiency can shed a lot of insight into immunodeficiency of HIV/AIDS.

Profound thymic atrophy with depletion of thymocytes and changes in thymic extracellular matrix are seen even in moderate malnutrition. It is however difficult to say whether these changes in thymic function are due to malnutrition *per se* or due to the severe infections frequently associated with malnutrition. Changes in thymic micro-environment like decreased thymic epithelial cells, expansion of extracellular matrix and decreased production of thymic hormone all contribute to thymic depletion. Thymocyte depletion results from increased apoptosis of CD4 and CD8 double-positive, double-negative and single-positive (immature) thymic lymphocytes. Apoptosis is driven by increased circulating levels of glucocorticoids, reduced leptin levels and deficiency of dietary protein and zinc.

Bone marrow cellularity is reduced, its stroma altered and there is limitation of extra-cellular matrix expansion. A study on bone marrow changes in children with PEM showed erythroid hypoplasia/dysplasia in the marrows of 50% children with kwashiorkor, 30% children with marasmic-kwashiorkor and 28.5% children with marasmus [114]. Suppression of cell cycle progression of haematopoietic progenitor cells with cell cycle arrest in G0/G1 phase is seen in protein malnutrition. This results in reduction in red cell and white cell lineages. In addition, bone marrow granulocytes display impaired blastic response to granulocyte-colony stimulating factor (G-CSF) and suboptimal mobilisation on lipopolysaccharide challenge. In protein-deficient mice models, bone marrow mesenchymal cells tend to differentiate into adipose cells, thereby altering the cytokine micro-environment in the bone marrow and compromising haematopoiesis. Despite this, the total number of leucocytes in peripheral blood of children with severe acute malnutrition remains normal. However, the number of dendritic cells is reduced [115]. Mice with transferrin receptor-1 deficiency are unable to absorb adequate iron. This results in impaired T-cell development and fewer mature B cells [116].

Secondary lymphoid tissue in the spleen and lymph nodes shows similar degenerative and hypo-proliferative changes in mouse protein-deficient models. The spleen has a thickened capsule and is deficient in splenocytes and splenic mononuclear cells. Cell cycle arrest, similar to that seen in the bone marrow, is seen. Splenic white pulp is also disorganised. Changes in lymph nodes can be seen even in moderate malnutrition. Zinc and iron deficiencies exaggerate changes caused by protein-energy malnutrition. There is hypoplasia of lymph nodes, decreased number of dendritic cells, macrophages, neutrophils and fibroblasts. The ability of lymph nodes to act as an effective barrier to pathogen spread is compromised. Poor trafficking of soluble antigens through the lymphoid conduits is also seen.

It would be intuitive to assume that like all other lymphoid tissue, the gut-associated lymphoid tissue (GALT) should also be hypoplastic in malnutrition. This has not been shown in humans conclusively.

5.1 Innate immune system dysfunction in malnutrition

Malnutrition affects the primary physical defensive barrier of the body. Thinning of dermis and reduced collagen levels are seen in animal models of PEM. In marasmic mice, thinning of the epidermis, with decreased hydration of stratum corneum, and decreased epidermal proliferation are seen. Wound healing is delayed and there is delayed wound contraction. Increased infiltration of wound site with inflammatory cells, decreased laying down of collagen, oedema of the extracellular matrix and altered neovascularisation are seen. Though skin changes like oedema and 'flaky paint dermatosis' and desquamation are common in kwashiorkor, there is no definite clinical proof to associate these changes with decreased immunity.

The changes in gut mucosa are more dramatic and have greater clinical consequences. These have been discussed above in environmental enteric dysfunction. At this juncture it suffices to say that gastric acid secretion is decreased in severe malnutrition, and gut permeability to bacteria is increased. In the oral cavity flow of saliva is reduced. Vitamin A deficiency reduces differentiation of epithelial cells in the skin, cornea and respiratory, urogenital and gastrointestinal tracts. This compromised epithelial barrier makes bacterial and viral invasion easy. Retinoic acid deficiency can alter gut mucosal barrier function. There is a marked reduction of type 3 innate lymphoid cells (ILC3) in gut mucosa of mice with vitamin A deficiency resulting in decreased production of IL-17 and Il-22 and increased susceptibility to bacterial infections. Concomitantly, there is an expansion of type 2 innate lymphoid cells (ILC2). These cells secrete IL-13 which causes goblet cell hyperplasia, increased mucus production and an increased resistance to gut helminths. Zinc reduces biofilm formation and decreases expression of virulence and adherence factors of entero-aggregative *Escherichia coli*. This may be one of the reasons for frequent diarrhoeal illnesses in malnourished children. A double-blinded randomised placebo controlled trial on zinc supplementation in children between the ages of 6 and 30 months in Delhi showed reduction in frequency, severity and duration of diarrhoea disease in the zinc-supplemented group [117].

Acute-phase reactant synthesis seems unaffected by malnutrition. C-reactive protein (CRP) rise is similar in normal and malnourished children when faced with an infectious challenge [118]. In contrast the so-called negative phase reactants like transferrin, pre-albumin, fibronectin and α2-HS glycoprotein are consistently decreased in malnutrition and do not rise adequately during an infectious challenge [119]. Complement levels are decreased in severe malnutrition. This is due to reduced synthesis in the liver and also increased consumption in the periphery. This is most marked in kwashiorkor. Reduction in C3 levels in malnutrition has been consistently reported from other studies as well [120].

As it has already been mentioned, there is no reduction in the total number of leucocytes in the peripheral blood. But chemotaxis and microbicidal activity of neutrophils are decreased in children with PEM. This may partly be due to decreased lysosomal enzyme synthesis and reduced glycolytic activity. Vitamin A is important for neutrophil maturation. Neutrophils in retinoic acid-deficient mouse models show impaired chemotaxis, phagocytosis and generation of reactive oxygen species. Vitamin A deficiency also decreases number and function of NK cells. Vitamin C deficiency in animals decreases apoptosis of neutrophils and results in their decreased clearance. Vitamin C deficiency exaggerates inflammation and retards its resolution in mouse model of sterile inflammation. Administration of vitamin C attenuates lung, kidney and liver injury in murine models of intra-abdominal sepsis and lethal LPS administration. The salutary effects of vitamin C in the lung include reduced pro-inflammatory response, increased epithelial barrier function, increased alveolar fluid clearance and decreased coagulopathy. Zinc modulates respiratory bursts in neutrophils. Moderate to severe malnutrition does not lead to reduction in absolute number of natural killer (NK) cells in children, but their function is depressed. Iron deficiency impairs macrophage function. Intracellular iron activates nuclear factor kB (NF kB). NfkB is responsible for exerting a restraint on reactive oxygen species and c-Jun-N-terminal kinase (JNK) signalling. These signalling pathways are crucial for antagonism of programmed cell death (PCD) induced by pro-inflammatory cytokines. Hypoxia-inducible factor-1α (HIF-1α) is an iron-dependent transcription factor that promotes synthesis of antimicrobial peptides by macrophages. Hence iron deficiency can lead to apoptosis of macrophages and also blunt their anti-microbial activity [121, 122].

Folate deficiency in rats is associated with reduced number of neutrophils and eosinophils. Zinc regulates release of pro-inflammatory cytokines like IL-1β, IL-6 and IFN-α by innate immune cells, and its deficiency leads to reduced synthesis of Th-1 cytokines. Selenium exerts its antioxidant activity via selenoproteins. They regulate pro-inflammatory mediators via mitogen-activated protein kinase and peroxisome proliferator-activated receptor-γ. Genetic knockout of selenoprotein genes in mice leads to impaired migration of macrophages and neutrophils and reduced phagocyte oxidative burst. Vitamin D plays a crucial role in macrophage function. Its deficiency increases risk of active TB and also increases risk of relapse of TB in both HIV-uninfected and HIV-positive individuals. The primary action of vitamin D is exerted via the vitamin D receptors on macrophages. There is a supplementary action via toll-like receptor signalling. Vitamin D leads to increased production of cathelicidin and β2-defensin which increase secretion of pro-inflammatory cytokines, induce anti-tuberculous autophagy and restrict growth of mycobacteria inside macrophages [123].

In severe malnutrition, dendritic cell numbers are reduced in peripheral blood and in lymphoid tissues. A study from Zambia showed reduced numbers of DCs and also impaired DC maturation and impaired ability of DCs to stimulated T-cell proliferation in the face of endotoxaemia. The DC function normalised with nutritional therapy [115]. Murine models with deficiency of protein, iron and zinc have shown reduction in number resident DCs in lymph nodes. These DCs also showed dysregulation of DC chemoattractants during inflammation. PEM grossly impairs antigen-presenting capacity and T-cell activation ability of DCs. Vitamin A, as retinoic acid, is vital for DC function. When there is inflammation, retinoic acid accelerates maturation and antigen-presenting capacity of DCs. Dendritic cells also store and release retinoic acid to act on other immune cells. Vitamin D plays an important role in regulation of DC function and exerts an anti-inflammatory role. It retards DC maturation, antigen presentation and T-cell priming.

5.2 Malnutrition and adaptive immune system

Malnutrition does not affect the total number of lymphocytes in peripheral blood. The total levels of immunoglobulins IgG and IgM in blood and secretory IgA in duodenal fluid and urine are unaltered. When malnutrition in children is compounded by a severe respiratory or intestinal bacterial infection, the number of B cells is reduced when compared to infected but well-nourished children. B lymphocyte function is preserved in PEM, but the profile of secreted immunoglobulins (Igs) and specific antibody-mediated immune responses are altered. Levels of Th1-type immunoglobulins (IgG2a and IgG3) are unaltered, those of tTh2-type Igs (IgG1 and IgE) are raised and those of secretory IgA are reduced. Severe protein malnutrition leads to decreased levels of secretory IgA in tears and saliva. Zinc deficiency depletes cells of B-cell lineage in the bone marrow. Vitamin A-deficient mice show a poor IgG response which is reversible by vitamin A supplementation. Vitamin A-deficient mice also have decreased number of IgA-secreting plasma cells in their Peyer's patches [123, 124].

Levels of CD4+ and CD8+ cells in peripheral blood remain unaltered in malnourished children hospitalised with serious infections. But there is a decrease in the number of CD4+ CD45RO+ memory T cells and effector T cells (CD4+ CD62L− and CD8+ CD28−) in severe malnutrition. Th1 cytokines required for Th1 differentiation (IL-7, IL-12, IL-18 and IL-21) and function (IL-2 and IFN-γ) are reduced in peripheral blood mononuclear cells of children with malnutrition and severe infection. In the same children, an overexpression of Th2 cytokines (IL-4 and IL-10) and increased apoptosis of CD3+ T cells is noted. The ability of T cells to respond to an inflammatory stimulus is also altered. There is an impaired antigen-specific T-cell response (decreased CD8+ cells and decreased IL-2 production by CD4+ cells), but antigen-specific antibody production is unimpaired. Proliferative response to phytohaemagglutinin is reduced. Delayed-type hypersensitivity response is also impaired in severe malnutrition. Zinc is required for Th1 differentiation and Th1 responses. It increases expression of IL-2, IFN-γ and IL-2Rb β2. Zinc deficiency therefore results in a reduction of CD4/CD8 ratio and levels of Th1 cytokines. Selenium deficiency adversely affects CD4+ T-cell proliferation, activation and function. The production of IL-2 and expression of IL-2 receptor are both reduced, and there is impaired mobilisation of calcium. Retinoic acid acts on naive T cells and promotes expression of gut-homing receptors, differentiation into Th2 phenotype and T-regulatory cells especially in the gut mucosa. It also inhibits maturation to Th1 phenotype or Th17 cells. RA activates B cells in mucosa and GALT to transform into IgA+ antibody secreting cells (ASC). Hence RA deficiency can seriously impair gut mucosal immunity. Due to its influence on effector T-cell function, vitamin A deficiency can lead to inadequate immune response to some vaccines. Vitamin A supplementation has been shown to lead to 20–30% reduction in all-cause mortality and reduction of incidence and severity diarrhoea diseases and measles [125, 126].

The effect of HIV infection on immune systems mirrors that of malnutrition in most aspects with just a few key differences. Natural killer cell activity and complement activity are increased in HIV infection. There is an increased secretion of pro-inflammatory cytokines (IL-1β, TNF-α, INF-γ and IL-6, IL-8 and soluble IL-2 receptors) and reduction of anti-inflammatory cytokines (IL-1 receptor antagonist, IL-4, IL-10 and IL-13). The chronic inflammatory state is also a hypercatabolic one and leads to increased mobilisation of amino acids from skeletal muscles that are further used for gluconeogenesis in the liver. TNF-α and IFN-γ also suppress appetite leading to decreased food intake. Hypercatabolism and decreased diet lead to malnutrition and HIV wasting. The combination of HIV and malnutrition aggravates reduction of CD4 and CD8 T cells, impairs bactericidal function of neutrophils and macrophages, impairs delayed-type hypersensitivity response and blunts antibody response to immunisation [97].

HIV infection also has a direct impact on nutrition. Studies have shown that among asymptomatic HIV-positive children, the rates of protein, carbohydrate and fat malabsorption are 30–60, 32 and 30%, respectively [127, 128]. Increased protein turnover occurs to cater for proliferation of neutrophils, fibroblasts and lymphocytes, production of immunoglobulins and acute-phase reactants and increased urinary nitrogen loss. This mainly comes from increased skeletal muscle breakdown and increased hepatic protein synthesis. Other metabolic changes that occur include elevated hepatic fatty acid synthesis, decreased peripheral lipoprotein lipase activity, hypertriglyceridemia, increased gluconeogenesis, insulin resistance and hyperglycaemia. There is redistribution of body stores of iron and zinc, with both being mobilised to the liver. This along with inadequate dietary intake leads to iron and zinc deficiencies. The pro-inflammatory state also leads to increased consumption of vitamins A, C and E which serve as antioxidants. There is reduction in levels of glutathione which is the principal intracellular antioxidant compound. Deficiencies of micronutrients like selenium, zinc, manganese and copper affect function of many key antioxidant enzymes. Deficiency of antioxidants leads to increased oxidative stress which triggers T-cell apoptosis and also enhances HIV replication [129].

6. Conclusion

Malnutrition depresses all aspects of immune function. HIV infection can lead to wasting and malnutrition by a complex interplay of aetiological factors. This malnutrition compounds immunodeficiency of AIDS and accelerates progression of disease and increases risk of mortality. Addressing nutrition right from the time of HIV diagnosis is a good strategy. Judicious and monitored nutritional therapy can mitigate NIADS and improve HIV clinical outcomes.

Author details

Vangal K. Sashindran[1*] and Rajneesh Thakur[2]

1 Internal Medicine, Armed Forces Medical Services, India, Prayagraj, India

2 Internal Medicine, Armed Forces Medical Services, India, Kanpur, India

*Address all correspondence to: vksashindran@gmail.com

IntechOpen

References

[1] Patel D, Bland R, Coovadia H, Rollins N, Coutsoudis A, Newell ML. Breastfeeding, HIV status and weights in South African children: A comparison of HIV-exposed and unexposed children. AIDS. 2010;**24**(3):437-445

[2] Nguefack F, Ehouzou MN, Kamgaing N, Chiabi A, Eloundou OE, Dongmo R, et al. Caractéristiques cliniques et évolutives de la malnutrition aiguë sévère chez les enfants infectés par le VIH: étude rétrospective sur 5 ans. Journal de Pédiatrie et de Puériculture. 2015;**28**(5):223-232

[3] Black RE, Allen LH, Bhutta ZA, Caulfield LE, De Onis M, Ezzati M, et al. Maternal and child undernutrition study group. Maternal and child undernutrition: Global and regional exposures and health consequences. The Lancet. 2008;**371**(9608):243-260

[4] International Food Policy Research Institute. Global Nutrition Report 2016. Washington, DC: International Food Policy Research Institute; 2016

[5] Black RE, Victora CG, Walker SP, Bhutta ZA, Christian P, De Onis M, et al. Maternal and child undernutrition and overweight in low-income and middle-income countries. The Lancet. 2013;**382**(9890):427-451

[6] Briend A, Khara T, Dolan C. Wasting and stunting—Similarities and differences: Policy and programmatic implications. Food and Nutrition Bulletin. 2015;**36**(Suppl 1):S15-S23

[7] Jesson J, Masson D, Adonon A, Tran C, Habarugira C, Zio R, et al. Prevalence of malnutrition among HIV-infected children in Central and West-African HIV-care programmes supported by the Growing Up Programme in 2011: A cross-sectional study. BMC Infectious Diseases. 2015;**15**(1):216

[8] Sewale Y, Hailu G, Sintayehu M, Moges NA, Alebel A. Magnitude of malnutrition and associated factors among HIV infected children attending HIV-care in three public hospitals in East and West Gojjam Zones, Amhara, Northwest, Ethiopia, 2017: A cross-sectional study. BMC Research Notes. 2018;**11**(1):788

[9] Agarwal D, Chakravarty J, Sundar S, Gupta V, Bhatia BD. Correlation between clinical features and degree of immunosuppression in HIV infected children. Indian Pediatrics. 2008;**45**(2):140

[10] Boettiger DC, Aurpibul L, Hudaya DM, Fong SM, Lumbiganon P, Saphonn V, et al. Antiretroviral therapy in severely malnourished, HIV-infected children in Asia. The Pediatric Infectious Disease Journal. 2016;**35**(5):e144

[11] UNICEF. WHO. World Bank. Joint child malnutrition estimates (UNICEF-WHO-WB)—Regional prevalence and numbers affected for wasting and severe wasting in 2013. 2015

[12] Andrade CS, Jesus RP, Andrade TB, Oliveira NS, Nabity SA, Ribeiro GS. Prevalence and characteristics associated with malnutrition at hospitalisation among patients with acquired immunodeficiency syndrome in Brazil. PLoS One. 2012;7(11):e48717

[13] Khalili H, Soudbakhsh A, Hajiabdolbaghi M, Dashti-Khavidaki S, Poorzare A, Saeedi AA, et al. Nutritional status and serum zing and selenium levels in Iranian HIV-infected individuals. BMC Infectious Diseases. 2008;**8**:165

[14] Mangili A, Murman DH, Zampini AM, Wanke CA. Nutrition and HIV infection: Review of weight loss and wasting in the era of highly active retroviral therapy from the nutrition for healthy living cohort. Clinical Infectious Diseases. 2006;**42**:836-842

[15] Ibrahim MK, Zambruni M, Melby CL, Melby PC. Impact of childhood malnutrition on host defense and infection. Clinical Microbiology Reviews. 2017;**30**(4):919-971

[16] Fergusson P, Tomkins A. HIV prevalence and mortality among children undergoing treatment for severe acute malnutrition in sub-Saharan Africa: A systematic review and meta-analysis. Transactions of the Royal Society of Tropical Medicine and Hygiene. 2009;**103**(6):541-548

[17] Rytter MJH, Kolte L, Briend A, Friis HChristensen VB. The immune system in children with malnutrition: A systematic review. PLoS One. 2014;**9**(8):e105017

[18] Tang AM, Forrester J, Spiegelman D, Knox TA, Tchetgen E, Gorbach SL. Weight loss and survival in HIV-positive patients in the era of highly active antiretroviral therapy. Journal of Acquired Immune Deficiency Syndromes. 2002;**31**(2):230-236

[19] Macallan DC, Noble C, Baldwin C, Jebb SA, Prentice AM, Coward WA, et al. Energy expenditure and wasting in human immunodeficiency virus infection. New England Journal of Medicine. 1995;**333**(2):83-88

[20] Powanda MC, Beisel WR. Metabolic effects of infection on protein and energy status. The Journal of Nutrition. 2003;**133**(1):322S-327S

[21] Melchior JC, Salmon D, Rigaud D, Leport C, Bouvet E, Detruchis P, et al. Resting energy expenditure is increased in stable, malnourished HIV-infected patients. The American Journal of Clinical Nutrition. 1991;**53**(2):437-441

[22] Grunfeld C, Pang M, Shimizu L, Shigenaga JK, Jensen P, Feingold KR. Resting energy expenditure, caloric intake, and short-term weight change in human immunodeficiency virus infection and the acquired immunodeficiency syndrome. The American Journal of Clinical Nutrition. 1992;**55**:455-460

[23] Shevitz AH, Knox TA, Spiegelman D, Roubenoff R, Gorbach SL, Skolnik PR. Elevated resting energy expenditure among HIV-seropositive persons receiving highly active antiretroviral therapy. AIDS. 1999;**13**:1351-1357

[24] Yarasheski KE, Zachwieja JJ, Gischler J, Crowley J, Horgan MM, Powderly WG. Increased plasma gln and Leu Ra and inappropriately low muscle protein synthesis rate in AIDS wasting. The American Journal of Physiology. 1998;**275**:E577-E583

[25] Macallan DC, McNurlan MA, Milne E, Calder AG, Garlick PJ, Griffin GE. Whole-body protein turnover from leucine kinetics and the response to nutrition in human immunodeficiency virus infection. The American Journal of Clinical Nutrition. 1995;**61**:818-826

[26] Roubenoff R, Grinspoon S, Skolnik PR. Role of cytokines and testosterone in regulating lean body mass and resting energy expenditure in HIV-infected men. American Journal of Physiology. Endocrinology and Metabolism. 2002;**283**:E138-E145

[27] Abad LW, Schmitz HR, Parker R, Roubenoff R. Cytokine responses differ by compartment and wasting status in patients with HIV infection and healthy controls. Cytokine. 2002;**18**:286-293

[28] Carr A, Cooper DA. Adverse effects of antiretroviral therapy. Lancet. 2000;**356**:1423-1430

[29] Lepik KJ, Yip B, Ulloa AC, Wang L, Toy J, Akagi L, et al. Adverse reactions to integrate strand transfer inhibitors. AIDS. 2018;**32**(7):903-912

[30] Rossit AR, Gonçalves AC, Franco C, Machado RL. Etiological agents of diarrhoea in patients infected by the human immunodeficiency virus-1: A review. Revista do Instituto de Medicina Tropical de São Paulo. 2009;**51**(2):59-65

[31] Krones E, Högenauer C. Diarrhoea in the immunocompromised patient. Gastroenterology Clinics. 2012;**41**(3):677-701

[32] Navin TR, Weber R, Vugia DJ, Rimland D, Roberts JM, Addiss DG, et al. Declining CD4+ T-lymphocyte counts are associated with increased risk of enteric parasitosis and chronic diarrhoea: Results of a 3-year longitudinal study. Journal of Acquired Immune Deficiency Syndromes and Human Retrovirology: Official Publication of the International Retrovirology Association. 1999;**20**(2):154-159

[33] Wuhib T, Silva TM, Newman RD, Garcia LS, Pereira ML, Chaves CS, et al. Cryptosporidial and microsporidial infections in human immunodeficiency virus-infected patients in northeastern Brazil. Journal of Infectious Diseases. 1994;**170**(2):494-497

[34] Goodgame RW. Understanding intestinal spore-forming protozoa: Cryptosporidia, microsporidia, isospora, and cyclospora. Annals of Internal Medicine. 1996;**124**(4):429-441

[35] Molina JM, Sarfati C, Beauvais B, Lémann M, Lesourd A, Ferchal F, et al. Intestinal microsporidiosis in human immunodeficiency virus-infected patients with chronic unexplained

diarrhoea: Prevalence and clinical and biologic features. Journal of Infectious Diseases. 1993;**167**(1):217-221

[36] Kotler DP, Orenstein JM. Prevalence of intestinal microsporidiosis in HIV-infected individuals referred for gastroenterological evaluation. American Journal of Gastroenterology. 1994;**89**(11):1998-2002

[37] Mnkemüller KE, Bussian AH, Lazenby A, Wilcox CM. Diarrhoea in human immunodeficiency virus infected patients: Where did all the microsporidia go. Gastroenterology. 1998;**114**:A1042

[38] Cegielski JP, Ortega YR, McKee S, Madden JF, Gaido L, Schwartz DA, et al. Cryptosporidium, Enterocytozoon, and Cyclospora infections in pediatric and adult patients with diarrhoea in Tanzania. Clinical Infectious Diseases. 1999;**28**(2):314-321

[39] Allason-Jones E, Mindel A, Sargeaunt P, Williams P. Entamoeba histolytica as a commensal intestinal parasite in homosexual men. New England Journal of Medicine. 1986;**315**(6):353-356

[40] Petri WA Jr, Singh U. Diagnosis and management of amebiasis. Clinical Infectious Diseases. 1999;**29**(5):1117-1125

[41] Haines CF, Moore RD, Bartlett JG, Sears CL, Cosgrove SE, Carroll K, et al. *Clostridium difficile* in a HIV-infected cohort: Incidence, risk factors, and clinical outcomes. AIDS. 2013;**27**(17):2799-2807

[42] Cello JP, Day LW. Idiopathic AIDS enteropathy and treatment of gastrointestinal opportunistic pathogens. Gastroenterology. 2009;**136**(6):1952-1965

[43] Zacharof A. AIDS-related diarrhoea—Pathogenesis,

evaluation and treatment. Annals of Gastroenterology. 2001;**14**(1):22-26

[44] Call SA, Heudebert G, Saag M, Wilcox CM. The changing etiology of chronic diarrhoea in HIV-infected patients with CD4 cell counts less than 200 cells/mm 3. The American Journal of Gastroenterology. 2000;**95**(11):3142

[45] Sun HY, Chen MY, Wu MS, Hsieh SM, Fang CT, Hung CC, et al. Endoscopic appearance of GI mycobacteriosis caused by the *Mycobacterium avium* complex in a patient with AIDS: Case report and review. Gastrointestinal Endoscopy. 2005;**61**(6):775-779

[46] Goodwin RA Jr, Shapiro JL, Thurman GH, Thurman SS, Des Prez RM. Disseminated histoplasmosis: Clinical and pathologic correlations. Medicine. 1980;**59**:1-33

[47] Rene E, Marche C, Chevalier T, Rouzioux C, Regnier B, Saimot AG, et al. Cytomegalovirus colitis in patients with acquired immunodeficiency syndrome. Digestive Diseases and Sciences. 1988;**33**(6):741-750

[48] Clerinx J, Bogaerts J, Taelman H, Habyarimana JB, Nyirabareja A, Ngendahayo P, et al. Chronic diarrhoea among adults in Kigali, Rwanda: Association with bacterial enteropathogens, rectocolonic inflammation, and human immunodeficiency virus infection. Clinical Infectious Diseases. 1995;**21**:1282-1284

[49] Grohmann GS, Glass RI, Pereira HG, Monroe SS, Hightower AW, Weber R, et al. Enteric viruses and diarrhoea in HIV-infected patients. Enteric Opportunistic Infections Working Group. New England Journal of Medicine. 1993;**329**:14-20

[50] Yan Z, Nguyen S, Poles M, Melamed J, Scholes JV. Adenovirus

colitis in human immunodeficiency virus infection: An underdiagnosed entity. The American Journal of Surgical Pathology. 1998;**22**:1101-1106

[51] Massimo F, Giovanna Z, Agata M, Loredana T, Paola M, Nicola P. Rotaviral infection and diarrhoea in health and HIV-infected children: A cohort study. Journal of Pediatric Gastroenterology & Nutrition. 1996;**23**(4):492-496

[52] Oshitani H, Kasolo FC, Mpabalwani M, Luo NP, Matsubayashi N, Bhat GH, et al. Association of rotavirus and human immunodeficiency virus infection in children hospitalized with acute diarrhoea, Lusaka, Zambia. Journal of Infectious Diseases. 1994;**169**(4):897-900

[53] Kotloff KL, Johnson JP, Nair P, Hickman D, Lippincott P, Wilson PD, et al. Diarrhoeal morbidity during the first 2 years of life among HIV-infected children. Journal of the American Medical Association. 1994;**271**(6):448-452

[54] Keiser PB, Nutman TB. Strongyloides stercoralis in the immunocompromised population. Clinical Microbiology Reviews. 2004;**17**(1):208-217

[55] DiBonaventura MD, Gupta S, Cho M, Mrus J. The association of HIV/AIDS treatment side effects with health status, work productivity, and resource use. AIDS Care. 2012;**24**(6):744-755

[56] Hill A, Balkin A. Risk factors for gastrointestinal adverse events in HIV treated and untreated patients. AIDS Reviews. 2009;**11**:30-38

[57] Braga Neto MB, Aguiar CV, Maciel JG. Evaluation of HIV protease and nucleoside reverse transcriptase inhibitors on proliferation, necrosis, apoptosis in intestinal epithelial cells and electrolyte and water transport and

epithelial barrier function in mice. BMC Gastroenterology. 2010;**10**:90

[58] Rufo PA, Lin PW, Andrade A, Jiang L, Rameh L, Flexner C, et al. Diarrhoea-associated HIV-1 APIs potentiate muscarinic activation of Cl-secretion by T84 cells via prolongation of cytosolic Ca^{2+} signaling. American Journal of Physiology-Cell Physiology. 2004;**286**(5):C998-C1008

[59] Bode H, Lenzner L, Kraemer OH, Kroesen AJ, Bendfeldt K, Schulzke JD, et al. The HIV protease inhibitors saquinavir, ritonavir, and nelfinavir induce apoptosis and decrease barrier function in human intestinal epithelial cells. Antiviral Therapy. 2005;**10**(5):645

[60] Wu X, Sun L, Zha W, Studer E, Gurley E, Chen L, et al. HIV protease inhibitors induce endoplasmic reticulum stress and disrupt barrier integrity in intestinal epithelial cells. Gastroenterology. 2010;**138**(1):197-209

[61] Brenchley JM, Douek DC. The mucosal barrier and immune activation in HIV pathogenesis. Current Opinion in HIV and AIDS. 2008;**3**(3):356

[62] Longstreth GF, Thompson WG, Chey WD, Houghton LA, Mearin F, Spiller RC. Functional bowel disorders. Gastroenterology. 2006;**130**:1480-1491

[63] Brandt LJ, Chey WD, Foxx-Orenstein AE, Schiller LR, Schoenfeld PS, Spiegel BM, et al. American College of Gastroenterology task force on irritable bowel syndrome. The American Journal of Gastroenterology. 2009;**104**(Suppl 1): S1-S35

[64] Batman PA, Miller AR, Forster SM, Harris JR, Pinching AJ, Griffin GE. Jejunal enteropathy associated with human immunodeficiency virus infection: Quantitative histology. Journal of Clinical Pathology. 1989;**42**(3):275-281

[65] Batman PA, Kotler DP, Kapembwa MS, et al. HIV enteropathy: Crypt stem and transit cell hyperproliferation induces villous atrophy in HIV/Microsporidia-infected jejunal mucosa. AIDS. 2007;**21**:433-439

[66] Keating J, Bjarnason I, Somasundaram S, Macpherson A, Francis N, Price AB, et al. Intestinal absorptive capacity, intestinal permeability and jejunal histology in HIV and their relation to diarrhoea. Gut. 1995;**37**(5):623-629

[67] Liu R, Huang L, Li J. HIV infection in gastric epithelial cells. The Journal of Infectious Diseases. 2013;**208**:1221-1230

[68] Maresca M, Mahfoud R, Garmy N, Kotler DP, Fantini J, Clayton F. The virotoxin model of HIV-1 enteropathy: Involvement of GPR15/Bob and galactosylceramide in the cytopathic effects induced by HIV-1 gp120 in the HT-29-D4 intestinal cell line. Journal of Biomedical Science. 2003;**10**(1):156-166

[69] Budge S, Parker AH, Hutchings PT, Garbutt C. Environmental enteric dysfunction and child stunting. Nutrition Reviews. 2019;**77**(4):240-253

[70] Kelly P, Besa E, Zyambo K, Louis-Auguste J, Lees J, Banda T, et al. Endomicroscopic and transcriptomic analysis of impaired barrier function and malabsorption in environmental enteropathy. PLoS Neglected Tropical Diseases. 2016;**10**(4):e0004600

[71] Marie C, Ali A, Chandwe K, Petri WA, Kelly P. Pathophysiology of environmental enteric dysfunction and its impact on oral vaccine efficacy. Mucosal Immunology. 2018;**9**:1

[72] Campbell DI, Elia M, Lunn PG. Growth faltering in rural Gambian infants is associated with impaired small intestinal barrier function, leading to endotoxemia and systemic

inflammation. The Journal of Nutrition. 2003;**133**(5):1332-1338

[73] Jacobs C, Chiluba C, Phiri C, Lisulo MM, Chomba M, Hill PC, et al. Seroepidemiology of hepatitis E virus infection in an urban population in Zambia: Strong association with HIV and environmental enteropathy. The Journal of Infectious Diseases. 2013;**209**(5):652-657

[74] Moniaci D, Greco D, Flecchia G, Raiteri R, Sinicco A. Epidemiology, clinical features and prognostic value of HIV-1 related oral lesions. Journal of Oral Pathology & Medicine. 1990;**19**(10):477-481

[75] Kolokotronis A, Kioses V, Antoniades D, Mandraveli K, Doutsos I, Papanayotou P. Immunologic status in patients infected with HIV with oral candidiasis and hairy leukoplakia. Oral Surgery, Oral Medicine, Oral Pathology. 1994;**78**(1):41-46

[76] Berberi A, Noujeim Z, Aoun G. Epidemiology of oropharyngeal candidiasis in human immunodeficiency virus/acquired immune deficiency syndrome patients and CD4+ counts. Journal of International Oral Health. 2015;**7**:20-23

[77] Swaminathan S, Padmapriyadarsini C, Sukumar B, Iliayas S, Kumar SR, Triveni C, et al. Nutritional status of persons with HIV infection, persons with HIV infection and tuberculosis, and HIV-negative individuals from southern India. Clinical Infectious Diseases. 2008;**46**(6):946-949

[78] Getahun H, Gunneberg C, Granich R, et al. HIV infection-associated tuberculosis: The epidemiology and the response. Clinical Infectious Diseases. 2010;**50**:S201-S207

[79] Corbett EL, Watt CJ, Walker N, Maher D, Williams BG, Raviglione MC, et al. The growing burden of tuberculosis: Global trends and interactions with the HIV epidemic. Archives of Internal Medicine. 2003;**163**(9):1009-1021

[80] Merchant RH, Lala MM. Common clinical problems in children living with HIV/AIDS: Systemic approach. The Indian Journal of Pediatrics. 2012;**79**(11):1506-1513

[81] Sinha U, Sengupta N, Mukhopadhyay P, Roy KS. Human immunodeficiency virus endocrinopathy. Indian Journal of Endocrinology and Metabolism. 2011;**15**(4):251

[82] Bornstein S. Predisposing factors for adrenal insufficiency. New England Journal of Medicine. 2009;**360**:2328-2339

[83] Zapanti E, Terzidis K, Chrousos G. Dysfunction of the hypothalamic-pituitary-adrenal axis in HIV infection and disease. Hormones. 2008;**7**(3):205-216

[84] Bhutta ZA, Das JK, Rizvi A. Evidence-based interventions for improvement of maternal and child nutrition: What can be done and at what cost? Lancet. 2013;**382**:452-477

[85] Trehan I, Goldbach HS, LaGrone LN. Antibiotics as part of the management of severe acute malnutrition. New England Journal of Medicine. 2013;**368**(5):425-435

[86] Chintu C, Bhat GJ, Walker AS. Co-trimoxazole as prophylaxis against opportunistic infections in HIV-infected Zambian children (CHAP): A double-blind randomised placebo-controlled trial. Lancet. 2004;**364**:1865-1871

[87] Bwakura-Dangarembizi M, Kendall L, Bakeera-Kitaka S. A randomized trial of prolonged co-trimoxazole in HIV-infected children in Africa. New England Journal of Medicine. 2014;**370**:41-53

[88] Church JA, Fitzgerald F, Walker AS, Gibb DM, Prendergast AJ. The expanding role of co-trimoxazole in developing countries. The Lancet Infectious Diseases. 2015;**15**:327-339

[89] Craig JC, Simpson JM, Williams GJ, Lowe A, Reynolds GJ, McTaggart SJ, et al. Antibiotic prophylaxis and recurrent urinary tract infection in children. New England Journal of Medicine. 2009;**361**(18):1748-1759

[90] Garly ML, Balé C, Martins CL, Whittle HC, Nielsen J, Lisse IM, et al. Prophylactic antibiotics to prevent pneumonia and other complications after measles: Community based randomised double blind placebo controlled trial in Guinea-Bissau. BMJ. 2006;**333**(7581):1245

[91] Aguilar C, Malphettes M, Donadieu J. Prevention of infections during primary immunodeficiency. Clinical Infectious Diseases. 2014;**59**:1462-1470

[92] Prendergast A, Walker AS, Mulenga V. Improved growth and anemia in HIV-infected African children taking cotrimoxazole prophylaxis. Clinical Infectious Diseases. 2011;**52**(7):953-956

[93] Jones KD, Thitiri J, Ngari M, Berkley JA. Childhood malnutrition: Toward an understanding of infections, inflammation, and antimicrobials. Food and Nutrition Bulletin. 2014;**35**(2_suppl 1):S64-S70

[94] Kim JH, Spiegelman D, Rimm E, Gorbach SL. The correlates of dietary intake among HIV-positive adults. The American Journal of Clinical Nutrition. 2001;**74**(6):852-861

[95] Piroth L, Duong M, Quantin C, Abrahamowicz M, Michardiere R, Aho LS, et al. Does hepatitis C virus co-infection accelerate clinical and immunological evolution of HIV-infected patients? AIDS. 1998;**12**(4):381-388

[96] Soriano V, Puoti M, Sulkowski M, Cargnel A, Benhamou Y, Peters M, et al. Care of patients coinfected with HIV and hepatitis C virus: 2007 updated recommendations from the HCV—HIV International Panel. AIDS. 2007;**21**(9):1073-1089

[97] Duggal S, Chugh TD, Duggal AK. HIV and malnutrition: Effects on immune system. Clinical and Developmental Immunology. 2012;**2012**:784740

[98] UNFAO. Declaration of the World Summit on Food Security. 2009

[99] Coates J, Swindale A, Bilinsky P. Household Food Insecurity Access Scale (HFIAS) for Measurement of Household Food Access: Indicator Guide (v. 3). Washington, DC: Food and Nutrition Technical Assistance Project, Academy for Educational Development; 2007

[100] Normén L, Chan K, Braitstein P, Anema A, Bondy G, Montaner JS, et al. Food insecurity and hunger are prevalent among HIV-positive individuals in British Columbia, Canada. The Journal of Nutrition. 2005;**135**:820-825

[101] Weiser SD, Fernandes KA, Brandson EK, Lima VD, Anema A, Bangsberg DR, et al. The association between food insecurity and mortality among HIV-infected individuals on HAART. Journal of Acquired Immune Deficiency Syndromes. 2009;**52**(3):342

[102] Benzekri NA, Sambou J, Diaw B, Sall EHI, Sall F, Niang A, et al. High prevalence of severe food insecurity and malnutrition among HIV-infected adults in Senegal, West Africa. PLoS ONE. 2015;**10**(11):e0141819

[103] Musumari PM, Wouters E, Kayembe PK, Nzita MK, Mbikayi SM,

Suguimoto SP, et al. Food insecurity is associated with increased risk of non-adherence to antiretroviral therapy among HIV-infected adults in the Democratic Republic of Congo: A cross-sectional study. PLoS One. 2014;**9**(1):e85327

[104] Hong SY, Fanelli TJ, Jonas A, Gweshe J, Tjituka F, Sheehan HM, et al. Household food insecurity associated with antiretroviral therapy adherence among HIV-infected patients in Windhoek, Namibia. Journal of Acquired Immune Deficiency Syndromes. 2014;**67**(4):e115-e122

[105] Mamlin J, Kimaiyo S, Lewis S, Tadayo H, Jerop FK, Gichunge C, et al. Integrating nutrition support for food-insecure patients and their dependents into an HIV care and treatment program in Western Kenya. American Journal of Public Health. 2009;**99**(2):215-221

[106] Tsai AC, Bangsberg DR, Emenyonu N, Senkungu JK, Martin JN, Weiser SD. The social context of food insecurity among persons living with HIV/AIDS in rural Uganda. Social Science & Medicine. 2011;**73**(12):1717-1724

[107] Hadgu TH, Worku W, Tetemke D, Berhe H. Undernutrition among HIV positive women in Humera hospital, Tigray, Ethiopia: Antiretroviral therapy alone is not enough, cross sectional study. BMC Public Health. 2013;**13**:943

[108] Foley W, Ward P, Carter P, Coveney J, Tsourtos G, Taylor A. An ecological analysis of factors associated with food insecurity in South Australia, 2002-7. Public Health Nutrition. 2010;**13**(2):215-221

[109] Laraia BA, Siega-Riz AM, Gundersen C, Dole N. Psychosocial factors and socioeconomic indicators are associated with household food insecurity among pregnant women. The Journal of Nutrition. 2006;**136**(1):177-182

[110] Bukusuba J, Kikafunda J, Whitehead R. Food security status in households of people living with HIV/AIDS (PLWHA) in a Ugandan urban setting. British Journal of Nutrition. 2007;**98**:211-217

[111] Ivers LC, Cullen KA, Freedberg KA, Block S, Coates J, Webb P, et al. HIV/AIDS, undernutrition, and food insecurity. Clinical Infectious Diseases. 2009;**49**(7):1096-1102

[112] Weiser S, Tuller D, Frongillo E, Senkungu J, Mukiibi N, Bangsberg D. Food insecurity as a barrier to sustained antiretroviral therapy adherence in Uganda. PLoS One. 2010;**5**(4):e10340

[113] Felicitee N, Seraphin N, Amamatou L, Njong TN, Roger D. Additional risk factors for malnutrition in children infected with HIV. JMR. 2018;**4**(2):63-68

[114] Ozkale M, Sipahi T. Hematologic and bone marrow changes in children with protein-energy malnutrition. Pediatric Hematology and Oncology. 2014;**31**:349-358

[115] Hughes SM, Amadi B, Mwiya M, Nkamba H, Tomkins A, Goldblatt D. Dendritic cell anergy results from endotoxemia in severe malnutrition. The Journal of Immunology. 2009;**183**(4):2818-2826

[116] Ned RM, Swat W, Andrews NC. Transferrin receptor 1 is differentially required in lymphocyte development. Blood. 2003;**102**(10):3711-3718

[117] Bhandari N, Bahl R, Taneja S, Strand T, Molbak K, Ulvik RJ, et al. Substantial reduction in severe diarrhoeal morbidity by daily zinc supplementation in young north Indian children. Pediatrics. 2002;**109**(6):e86

[118] Malavé I, Vethencourt MA, Pirela M, Cordero R. Serum levels of thyroxine-binding prealbumin, C-reactive protein and interleukin-6 in protein-energy undernourished children and normal controls without or with associated clinical infections. Journal of Tropical Pediatrics. 1998;**44**(5):256-262

[119] Yoder MC, Anderson DC, Gopalakrishna GS, Douglas SD, Polin RA. Comparison of serum fibronectin, prealbumin, and albumin concentrations during nutritional repletion in protein-calorie malnourished infants. Journal of Pediatric Gastroenterology and Nutrition. 1987;**6**(1):84-88

[120] Haller L, Zubler RH, Lambert PH. Plasma levels of complement components and complement haemolytic activity in protein-energy malnutrition. Clinical and Experimental Immunology. 1978;**34**(2):248

[121] Bubici C, Papa S, Dean K, Franzoso G. Mutual cross-talk between reactive oxygen species and nuclear factor-kappa B: Molecular basis and biological significance. Oncogene. 2006;**25**(51):6731

[122] Chen L, Xiong S, She H, Lin SW, Wang J, Tsukamoto H. Iron causes interactions of TAK1, p21ras, and phosphatidylinositol 3-kinase in caveolae to activate IκB kinase in hepatic macrophages. Journal of Biological Chemistry. 2007;**282**(8):5582-5588

[123] Ibrahim MK, Zambruni M, Melby CL, Melby PC. Impact of childhood malnutrition on host defence and infection. Clinical Microbiology Reviews. 2017;**30**(4):919-971

[124] Mora JR, Iwata M, von Andrian UH. Vitamin effects on the immune system: Vitamins A and D take centre stage. Nature Reviews.

Immunology. 2008;**8**:685-698. DOI: 10.1038/nri2378

[125] Imdad A, Mayo-Wilson E, Herzer K, Bhutta ZA. Vitamin A supplementation for preventing morbidity and mortality in children from six months to five years of age. Cochrane Database of Systematic Reviews. 2017 Mar 11;**3**(3):CD008524. DOI: 10.1002/14651858

[126] Awasthi S, Peto R, Read S, Clark S, Pande V, Bundy D. DEVTA (deworming and enhanced vitamin A) team. Vitamin A supplementation every 6 months with retinol in 1 million pre-school children in North India: DEVTA, a cluster-randomised trial. The Lancet. 2013;**381**(9876):1469-1477

[127] Yolken RH, Hart W, Oung I, Shiff C, Greenson J, Perman JA. Gastrointestinal dysfunction and disaccharide intolerance in children infected with human immunodeficiency virus. The Journal of Pediatrics. 1991;**118**(3):359-363

[128] Guarino A, Albano F, Tarallo L, Castaldo A, Rubino A, Borgia G, et al. Intestinal malabsorption of HIV-infected children: Relationship to diarrhoea, failure to thrive, enteric micro-organisms and immune impairment. AIDS. 1993;7(11):1435-1440

[129] Kalebic T, Kinter A, Poli G, Anderson ME, Meister A, Fauci AS. Suppression of human immuno-deficiency virus expression in chronically infected monocytic cells by glutathione, glutathione ester, and N-acetylcysteine. Proceedings of the National Academy of Sciences of the United States of America. 1991;**88**(3):986

Chapter 4

Nutrition Habits in People Living with HIV/AIDS in Bulgaria: Review of Current Practice and Recommendations

Maria Jordanova Dimitrova

Abstract

The innovations in the medical science and development of new biotechnology medicines changed significantly the course of the human immune-deficiency virus (HIV) infection toward a chronic condition. Along HAART, habits in nutrition place an important role in the improvement of the health status of people living with HIV. Proper diet and nutrition may enhance the adherence and concordance to prescribed therapy and its effectiveness, to reduce the risk of adverse drug events and to boost the immune function. In the resent years a tendency towards increased food supplements consumption is observed, especially in patients with chronic diseases. There is a risk of possible interactions between selected dietary supplements with the antiretroviral medicines which may result in decrease of the drug concentrations in the blood plasma and subsequent decreased therapeutic effect and increased risk of viral resistance. Still there are gaps in respect with such information in the guidelines and recommendations for treatment, monitoring and nutrition in HIV. More studies are needed to fully evaluate such interactions and to put recommendations both for the healthcare professionals and for the people living with HIV for their use in order not to compromise HAART and to maintain the desirable therapeutic outcome.

Keywords: HIV, nutrition, food supplements, highly active antiretroviral therapy, interactions

1. Introduction

The innovations in the medical science and development of new biotechnology medicines changed significantly the course of the human immune-deficiency virus (HIV) infection towards a chronic condition. The advancement of the highly active antiretroviral therapy (HAART) led to significant increase in the life expectancy allowing people living with HIV to have a near-normal life-expectancy while meeting a variety of acute and chronic care needs [1].

Along HAART, nutrition habits place an important role in the improvement of the health status of people living with HIV. Proper diet and nutrition (food-based attitude and micronutrient supplementation) may enhance the adherence and concordance to prescribed therapy and its effectiveness, to reduce the risk of adverse drug events and to boost the immune function. On the other side, one of the main concerns in terms of nutrition habits, especially food supplement intake, is related to possible interactions with the antiretroviral medicines which may result in decrease of the drug concentrations in the blood plasma and subsequent decreased therapeutic effect and increased risk of viral resistance [2]. In this respect there are still gaps of scientific evidence for the antiretroviral drug-to-supplement interactions and only a few dietary supplements (i.e., Ca, Mg, Fe supplements) have been evaluated in combination with the currently available on the pharmaceutical market antiretroviral medicines [3, 4]. While, there is a tendency towards increased consumption of food supplements among patients with chronic diseases, healthcare providers should monitor their patients for potentially important drug—supplement interactions. People living with HIV should also be willing to communicate with their healthcare providers any administration of dietary supplements and special nutrition regimes in order to optimize their intake in compliance with the prescribed HAART and to avoid possible undesirable interactions.

It is a matter of national practices of the competent authorities and healthcare providers to provide reliable knowledge and adequate nutrition habits in people living with HIV to assure increased compliance and to maintain the effectiveness of the therapy.

2. Nutrition recommendations and habits of people living with HIV

In the recent years a tendency towards optimization of the HAART due to the development of new drug formulations, including fixed dose combinations led to decease in the "pill burden" and increase in the tolerability due to better safety profile [5]. Improvements in the drug supply process led to better access to HAART. Along with this there are growing evidences for the influence of lifestyle habits and nutrition on onset and progression of different chronic and socially important diseases. Due to these reasons nutrition recommendations and guidelines are created to help the competent national authorities, healthcare providers and people living with HIV to create overall care plan.

Literature search of published recommendations and habits for nutrition and HIV was performed in the scientific databases PubMed, Google Scholar, Scopus, Research gate using key words—nutrition, recommendations, guidelines, HIV.

2.1 Nutrition recommendations

Literature search aimed to find and review the scope and recommendations in published guides and scientific manuscripts for nutrition and HIV.

2.1.1 Guidelines for nutrition and HIV

Since 2002, the World Health Organization has issued a set of guidelines and manuals on nutritional care and support for people living with HIV/AIDS, nutrient requirements, regional consultations on nutrition, and integrated approaches to nutritional care of HIV-infected children [6–8].

The main scope of these guidelines and manuals is to promote proper nutrient requirements in people living with HIV and to focus on the need of adequate nutrition and access to food in all regions, especially in the developing countries. The guidelines give detailed information on the recommended daily intake of different micronutrients (i.e., vitamin A, C and E and B-complex vitamins, iron-folate supplementation, to boost the immune system and to meet the increased energy requirements of people living with HIV, sets of recommendations for appropriate food intake and the importance of the type of food for the effect of the antiretroviral therapy [9].

The WHO guides recommend that all national health authorities should provide counseling on the management of the long-term nutritional aspects of the antiretroviral therapies. It is also recommended that healthcare providers should improve the attention of people living with HIV that diet and nutrition may enhance the acceptability of their prescribed HAART and to improve adherence and effectiveness of therapy.

In 2001, a guide for nutrition care and support in HIV/AIDS was published thanks to the Food and Nutrition Technical Assistance Project of the Office of Health, Infectious Disease and Nutrition and the Bureau for Global Health at the US Agency for International Agreement. This document provided guidance on general nutrition care and support of people living with HIV, the role and source of selected micronutrients [10]. In 2004, this report was updated with information concerning mainly different types of important drug-drug interactions, food-medication interactions, and their impact on the effect of the antiretroviral therapy and detailed recommendations on how to avoid such interactions depending on the prescribed antiretroviral medicines. The guide also focuses on the need to identify reliable sources (i.e., Ministries of health, drug product information, pharmaceutical services, journals and patient organizations) of easy to comprehend information in the light of improved access to existing and new antiretroviral medicines, possible important drug-drug and drug-food/food supplement interactions [11].

In their latest updates the Guidelines of the U.S. Department of Health and Human Services and of the European AIDS Clinical society (v.9.1) for the treatment and monitoring of HIV/AIDS set list of recommendations and cautions possible interactions and effects between food and Ca, Mg and Fe supplements with the antiretroviral medicines [12, 13]. The guidelines also focus that the healthcare providers should always monitor their patients in terms of any food supplement intake for possible interactions with their prescribed HAART, not only in case of therapeutic failure.

2.1.2 Published articles for nutrition recommendation

The guidelines on treatment, monitoring and nutrition and HIV discussed above put more focus on the needs for adequate and proper nutrition and give practical advices for dietary regimes and micronutrient daily needs. Special focus is put also on the interactions between food and Ca, Mg and Fe supplements and antiretroviral medicines interactions.

However, there are still gaps of information in the guidelines concerning possible interactions between some food supplements, containing herbal products (i.e., St. John's wort, *Echinacea*, ginkgo) and the antiretroviral medicines and their impact on the therapeutic effect. For this reason the second part of the literature search focused on recommendations on nutrition and HIV from published scientific articles evaluating this type of interactions.

Results from systematic review published in 2017 show that the most frequently reported food supplement-antiretroviral medicine interactions in the literature from herbal origin are with St. John wort, ginkgo, milk thistle and cat's claw [14]. The proposed mechanism of action was examined mostly in pharmacokinetic studies and case-reports. It is considered that most probably these food supplements interact with the antiretroviral medicines on CYP450 enzyme system level either inhibiting or inducing different CYP 540 enzymes thus causing adverse events or reduced therapeutic response respectively. In the systematic review are included also studies evaluating the interactions between some micronutrients like vitamin C, ferrous fumarate, calcium carbonate, zinc sulfate and multivitamin. The latter are considered to form chelation with entry inhibitors (maraviroc), integrase inhibitors (dolutegravir, raltegravir), protease inhibitors (atazanavir, darunavir, lopinavir, ritonavir, etc.), non-nucleoside reverse transcriptase inhibitors (efavirenz, etravirine) and nucleoside reverse transcriptase inhibitors (abacavir, emtricitabine, lamivudine, tenofovir) thus causing reduction in the therapeutic effect. The systematic review found also that for some of the dietary supplements there were controversial results but statistically significant interactions with selected antiretrovirals were found for St. John's wort, vitamin C, zinc sulfate, ferrous fumarate, calcium carbonate, multivitamins and some forms of ginkgo, garlic, and milk thistle [4, 15–17]. With this respect people living with HIV, who are prescribed HAART, should better avoid taking them. Cat's claw and evening primrose oil are found to increase significantly the levels of selected antiretrovirals and close monitoring for adverse effects is recommended [18, 19].

2.1.3 Nutrition guidelines and recommendations in Bulgaria

Bulgaria is a country with low HIV infection prevalence in the general population (2.8 per 100,000) but still there is a risk of rapid spread of epidemics in certain "most-at-risk" groups-injecting drug use and sex between men. There is already an epidemiological evidence for these groups and the main concern is the possibility of transmission of the infection to the general population [20]. In the resent years there is also a tendency in increase in the transmission via heterosexual contact (39% for 2016). The most affected age group is 30–39 years and the number of man is almost five times higher than the women [21].

In 2016, the Ministry of Health published two methodology guides - one for antiretroviral treatment and monitoring of adult people living with HIV. The guidance is based on the European guidelines for treatment and monitoring of HIV of the European AIDS Clinical Society from 2015 and gives straightforward recommendations and cautions for interactions between food and Ca, Mg and Al containing anti-acid medicine with selected available on the pharmaceutical market antiretroviral medicines and recommendations to the healthcare professionals to pay attention to possible drug-food and drug-food supplement interactions in case of treatment failure [22]. The other is a methodology guidance on prophylaxis of HIV transmission from mother to child was also published. This guidance gives nutrition recommendations for the children [23].

2.2 Nutrition habits

Nutrition habits and lifestyle play an important role in the overall care process of different chronic diseases and can contribute to the compliance to the prescribed pharmacotherapy [24].

Healthy diet, physical activity and proper micronutrient supplementation consistent with HAART can boost immune response, reduce side effect of medicines, improve the health status and can help people living with HIV to adhere better to therapy.

Studies have shown that people living with HIV tend to use dietary supplements as a part of their treatment care plan – mostly antioxidants and supplements from herbal origin. These patients are also more likely to use internet for searching and sharing health-related information. This hides a risk of misinformation from non-reliable sources of health information [25].

Competent healthcare authorities together with different non-profit and patients' organizations have developed online sources for health information with advices for nutrition habits, healthy lifestyle and dietary regimes [26–28].

Most of these sources of information, however, focus on the importance of nutrition, pay attention on the daily micronutrient intake, energy consumption and provide ready dietary recipes. Still there is lack of information concerning the concordance of different micronutrient supplements with the prescribed antiretroviral therapy.

An ongoing study in Bulgaria among people living with HIV and their healthcare providers is evaluating the tendency for utilization of dietary supplements, the knowledge for possible dietary supplements-drug interactions and the sources of respective health-related information.

Preliminary results show that 50% of the people living with HIV, participating in the inquiry, are following healthy lifestyle including active physical activity and dietary regimes rich in proteins, fats and vegetables. Half of the inquired use dietary supplements mostly are proteins, amino-acids, vitamin C, vitamin D, fatty acids and multivitamins.

About 88% of the inquired agree that the balanced healthy dietary regime is important to boost the immune system and are aware of possible interactions between the prescribed therapy and the dietary supplements they are taking, 62% believe that the nutrition is important for HAART adherence.

The preliminary results also show that people living with HIV tend to use internet for health related source of information—86% use internet as a main source of information concerning nutrition and its impact on the health status and prescribed therapy. About 71% of these patients rely mostly on the information presented on the websites of patients' organizations.

The healthcare providers follow the methodology guidance for treatment and monitoring of adult people living with HIV issued by the Ministry of health. They also pay attention to the people living with HIV who are prescribed HAART not to take St. John's wort and ginkgo due to negative impact on the therapeutic effect of the antiretroviral medicines.

These preliminary results are consistent with those found in the literature and show the increasing tendency of administration of food supplements and the related with this search of health related information in internet.

3. Practical advices for nutrition and HIV for the Bulgarian health care setting

3.1 Practical advices for use of dietary supplements

The review of literature shows that the Bulgarian methodology guidance for treatment and monitoring of HIV in adult people is consistent with the European guidelines but since 2016, it has not been updated. The latest version (9.1) of the European guidelines for treatment and monitoring of HIV in adults gives information for some possible interactions between the antiretrovirals and Ca, Mg, and Fe supplements and multivitamins.

Based on this and the preliminary results from the inquiry, the advices for use of dietary supplements, which interact with available on the Bulgarian pharmaceutical market antiretrovirals, could be summarized in the following table (**Table 1**).

It should be noted that the European guidelines for treatment and monitoring of HIV in adults give detailed information on the potent interactions between micronutrients and particular HAART regime, while those interactions published in the literature from pharmacokinetic and case-report studies are only for selected antiretrovirals. That is way when healthcare professionals evaluate the risks of possible interactions should consider each of the antiretrovirals included in the HAART. For those possible interactions between medicines and food supplements for which an advice for use in concordance with HAART or recommendation for

Dietary supplement	Antiretrovirals	Potential outcome	Caution	Source
Micronutrient supplements				
Multivitamins and Al/Ca/Mg supplements	Dolutegravir/abacavir/lamivudine	Reduced therapeutic effect	Take separate in time (2 h after or 6 h before)	[14]
Multivitamins and Al/Ca/Mg supplements	Tenofovir disoproxil fumarate/ emtricitabine, tenofovir alafenamide/ emtricitabine	Reduced therapeutic effect	Take separate in time (2 h after of 6 h before)	[14]
Multivitamins and Al/Ca/Mg supplements	Dolutegravir	Reduced therapeutic effect	Take separate in time (2 h after of 6 h before)	[14]
Multivitamins and Al/Ca/Mg supplements and high doses Ca	Raltegravir 1200 mg once daily	Reduced therapeutic effect	Not recommended. Instead administer raltegravir 400 mg twice daily	[14]
Zinc sulfate	Efavirenz, etravirine, raltegravir, dolutegravir, abacavir, emtricitabine, tenofovir, zidovudine, lamivudine	Reduced therapeutic effect	Chelation suspected	[15]
Vitamin C	Atazanavir, darunavir, fosamprenavir, lopinavir, ritonavir, saquinavir, efavirenz, etravirine, dolutegravir	Reduced therapeutic effect	CYP3A4 induction suspected	[15]
Dietary supplements of herbal origin—potential CYP3A4 induction mechanism				
St John's wort	Atazanavir, darunavir, fosamprenavir, lopinavir, ritonavir, saquinavir, efavirenz, dolutegravir	Reduced therapeutic effect	CYP3A4 induction	[15]
Ginkgo	Atazanavir, darunavir, fosamprenavir, lopinavi, ritonavir, saquinavir, efavirenz, etravirine, dolutegravir	Reduced therapeutic effect	CYP3A4 induction	[15]
Garlic	Atazanavir, darunavir, fosamprenavir, lopinavir, ritonavir, saquinavir	Reduced therapeutic effect	CYP3A4 induction	[15]
Milk thistle	Atazanavir, darunavir, fosamprenavir, lopinavir, ritonavir, saquinavir, efavirenz, etravirine, dolutegravir	Reduced therapeutic effect	CYP3A4 induction	[15]
Dietary supplements of herbal origin—potential CYP3A4 inhibition mechanism				
Cat's claw	Atazanavir, darunavir, fosamprenavir, lopinavir, ritonavir, saquinavir, efavirenz, etravirine, dolutegravir	Adverse effects	CYP3A4 inhibition	[15]
Evening primrose Oil	Atazanavir, darunavir, fosamprenavir, lopinavir, ritonavir, saquinavir, efavirenz, etravirine, dolutegravir	Adverse effects	CYP3A4 and CYP2D6 inhibition	[15]

Table 1.
Potential interactions between antiretrovirals and micronutrients and dietary supplements of herbal origin available on the Bulgarian pharmaceutical market.

no use at all is not reported yet, it is advisable healthcare professionals and people living with HIV should monitor for possible effects on the therapeutic outcome and for adverse events.

As the national guidance is not updated in the same pace as the international ones it is recommendable healthcare professionals to be up-to-date with the most current recommendations and guidelines.

It is advisable people living with HIV to communicate with their healthcare professionals possible use of dietary supplements and micronutrients in order to not to interfere negatively with their prescribed therapy.

3.2 Practical advices for use of health-related sources of information

The preliminary results from the inquiry show that people living with HIV are more likely to use internet health-care related sources of information related to nutrition and lifestyle. In this respect, in order to prevent misinformation, it is advisable to recognize reliable sources like websites of the patients' organizations and trusted health websites. Most of these websites, however, do not present information about drug-drug and drug-micronutrient and dietary supplement information. That is way it is advisable that people living with HIV to communicate with their healthcare providers the nutrition and lifestyle habits as well. Healthcare professionals can discuss with them trusted sources of health-related information and recommend such.

4. Discussion

The literature search on the nutrition habits and HIV shows that the competent health authorities worldwide consistently issue recommendations and guidelines which could be implemented on national level.

On the basis of the increased need for healthy lifestyle as an important component of the treatment process of many chronic diseases and the increased consumption of food supplements [29], more studies with higher significance of the results should be performed in order to fully evaluate the possible interactions between different medicines and available food supplements and micronutrients.

The study on the current practice on nutrition habits and HIV in Bulgaria shows that people living with HIV acknowledge the importance of nutrition and healthy lifestyle for the adherence and the overall effect of the antiretroviral therapy and the majority of them are informed about possible interactions between the prescribed antiretroviral therapy and the dietary supplements and micronutrients they are taking, mostly from internet. These results are consistent with those published in the literature.

The study has this limitation that the current results are preliminary as it is still ongoing.

The Bulgarian guidelines for treatment and monitoring of HIV in adults are consistent with the European ones but are not updated and the same pace and currently do not give information on food supplement-drug interactions. However, they recommend that healthcare professionals should be aware of such in case of treatment failure.

Patients' organizations in Bulgaria are very active and maintain up-to-date websites and other sources of information like brochures and periodic initiatives and meetings but still there is a lack of information about the potent interactions between drugs and dietary supplements in the light of increased consumption of food supplements in the overall population [30].

It is advisable that people living with HIV communicate more with their healthcare professionals in respect to their nutrition habits in order not to compromise the therapeutic effect of their prescribed therapy.

5. Conclusion

The innovations in the medical science and development of new biotechnology medicines changed the course of the human immune-deficiency virus (HIV) infection towards a chronic condition and increased significantly the life expectance.

People living with HIV are more likely to follow healthy lifestyle and build proper nutrition habits but are also willing to use food supplements and micronutrients as a part of their care plan. They acknowledge that nutrition habits place an important role in the improvement of the health status, enhance the adherence and concordance to prescribed therapy and its effectiveness, reduction in the risk of adverse drug events and to boost the immune function. However, there is a risk of possible interactions with the antiretroviral medicines which may result in decrease of the drug concentrations in the blood plasma and subsequent decreased therapeutic effect and increased risk of viral resistance.

International guidelines are issued periodically to help competent health authorities and healthcare professions in the process of care of people living with HIV. The guidelines for treatment and monitoring of HIV in adults and those for nutrition and HIV already present information about potent interactions between selected micronutrients and antiretrovirals, but still there are gaps of information concerning possible interactions between drugs and food supplements from herbal origin.

People living with HIV are also more likely to use internet for nutrition and health-related sources of information. In this light competent authorities, healthcare professionals and patients' organizations should place info-vigilance strategies to monitor the reliability of health-related information in order to protect consumers from misinformation. People should be advised to use only trusted medical websites and have closer communication with their healthcare professionals. They should be also educated how to monitor their health status and what possible outcomes to expect when using food supplements and micronutrients (desirable or negative) alongside the prescribed antiretroviral therapy and should always communicate with their healthcare professionals (physicians and pharmacists) any changes in their nutrition habits. Healthcare professionals should follow the most up-to-date recommendations in order to individualize and assure proper nutrition habits as a part of the total treatment plan of people living with HIV.

More studies are needed to fully evaluate the possible interactions between the different medicines and available food supplements and micronutrients and propose mechanism of action in order not to optimize and not to compromise the desired therapeutic outcomes.

Acknowledgements

I would like to thank professor Guenka Petrova for her help, empathy and guidance in my every-day academic and scientific work, to professor Radka Argirova and professor George Momekov for their highly appreciated expertise, and to all healthcare professionals and people living with HIV who showed willingness to participate in the inquiry.

Conflict of interest

The author declares no conflict of interest.

Author details

Maria Jordanova Dimitrova
Department of Organization and Economy of Pharmacy, Faculty of Pharmacy,
Medical University of Sofia, Sofia, Bulgaria

*Address all correspondence to: mia_dimitrova@yahoo.com

IntechOpen

References

[1] Ettner SL, Conover CJ, Proescholdbell RJ, Weaver MR, Ang A, Arno PS. AIDS Care. 2008;**20**(10):1177-1189

[2] Hermann R, von Richter O. Clinical evidence of herbal drugs as perpetrators of pharmacokinetic drug interactions. Planta Medica. 2012;**78**:1458-1477

[3] Moltó J, Valle M, Miranda C, et al. Herb-drug interaction between *Echinacea purpurea* and etravirine in HIV-infected patients. Antimicrobial Agents and Chemotherapy. 2012;**56**:5328-5331

[4] Moyle G, Else L, Jackson A, et al. Coadministration of atazanavir-ritonavir and zinc sulfate: Impact on hyperbilirubinemia and pharmacokinetics. Antimicrobial Agents and Chemotherapy. 2013;**57**:3640-3644

[5] Nachega JB, Parienti JJ, Uthman OA, Gross R, Dowdy DW, et al. Lower pill-burden and once-daily antiretroviral treatment regimens for HIV infection: A meta-analysis of randomized controlled trials. Clinical Infectious Diseases. 2014;**58**(9):1297-1307. DOI: https://doi.org/10.1093/cid/ciu046

[6] World Health Organization. Living Well with HIV/AIDS: A Manual on Nutrition Care and Support for People Living with HIV/AIDS. Available from: https://www.who.int/nutrition/publications/hivaids/y4168E00.pdf?ua=1. [Accessed: 10 November 2018]

[7] World Health Organization. Regional Consultation on nutrition and HIV/AIDS: Evidence, lessons and recommendations for action in South-East Asia 2007. Available from: https://www.who.int/nutrition/publications/hivaids/Regional_consultation_NUTHIV_SEA.pdf?ua=1 [Accessed: 20 November 2018]

[8] WHO Guidelines on HIV and Infant Feeding 2010. An Updated Framework for Priority Action. Available from: http://apps.who.int/iris/bitstream/handle/10665/75152/FWC_MCA_12.1_eng.pdf?sequence=1. [Accessed: 25 November 2018]

[9] World Health Organization. Nutrient Requirements for People Living with HIV/AIDS: Report of a Technical Consultation. 2003. Available from: http://apps.who.int/iris/bitstream/handle/10665/42853/9241591196.pdf?ua=1. [Accessed: 15 November 2018]

[10] HIV/AIDS: A Guide for Nutrition, Care and Support. Food and Nutrition Technical Assistance Project. Washington DC: Academy for Educational Development; 2001

[11] HIV/AIDS: A Guide For Nutritional Care and Support. 2nd Edition. Food and Nutrition Technical Assistance Project, Washington DC: Academy for Educational Development; 2004

[12] Panel on Antiretroviral Guidelines for Adults and Adolescents. Guidelines for the Use of Antiretroviral Agents in Adults and Adolescents Living with HIV. Department of Health and Human Services. Available from: http://www.aidsinfo.nih.gov/ContentFiles/AdultandAdolescentGL.pdf. [Accessed: 30 November 2018]

[13] European AIDS Clinical Society. European Guidelines for Treatment of HIV-Positive Adults in Europe. Available from: http://www.eacsociety.org/files/2018_guidelines-9.1-english.pdf. [Accessed: 30 November 2018]

[14] Jalloh MA, Gregory PJ, Hein D, Cochrane ZR, Rodriguez A. Dietary supplement interactions with antiretrovirals: A systematic review. International Journal of STD & AIDS. 2017;**28**(1):4-15

[15] Song I, Borland J, Arya N, et al. Pharmacokinetics of dolutegravir when administered with mineral supplements in healthy adult subjects. Journal of Clinical Pharmacology. 2015;**55**:490-496

[16] Piscitelli SC, Burstein AH, Welden N, et al. The effect of garlic supplements on the pharmacokinetics of saquinavir. Clinical Infectious Diseases. 2002;**34**:234-238

[17] Slain D, Amsden JR, Khakoo RA, et al. Effect of highdose vitamin C on the steady-state pharmacokinetics of the protease inhibitor indinavir in healthy volunteers. Pharmacotherapy. 2005;**25**:165-170

[18] López Galera RM, Ribera Pascuet E, Esteban Mur JI, et al. Interaction between cat's claw and protease inhibitors atazanavir, ritonavir and saquinavir. European Journal of Clinical Pharmacology. 2008;**64**:1235-1236

[19] Beukel van den Bout-van den CJ, Bosch ME, Burger DM, et al. Toxic lopinavir concentrations in an HIV-1 infected patient taking herbal medications. AIDS. 2008;**22**:1243-1244

[20] Dimitrova M, Petrova G, Manova M, Savova A, Yancheva N, et al. Economic impact of the highly active antiretroviral pharmacotherapy on cost and HIV/AIDS control in Bulgaria. Biotechnology & Biotechnological Equipment; **2012**. DOI: 10.5504/BBEQ.2012.0076

[21] National Program for Prevention and Control of HIV/AIDS, Ministry of Health. Available from: http://www.aidsprogram.bg/information1-%D0%9F%D0%BE%D1%81%D0%BB%D0%B5%D0%B4%D0%BD%D0%B8%20%D0%B4%D0%B0%D0%BD%D0%BD%D0%B8%20%D0%B7%D0%B0%20%D0%A1%D0%9F%D0%98%D0%9D%20%D0%B2%2%D0%91%D1%8A%D0%BB%D0%B3%D0%B0%D1%

80%D0%B8%D1%8F-312-bg.html. [Accessed: 10 November 2018]

[22] Methodology Guidance on Antiretroviral Treatment and Monitoring of Adult with; HIV in Bulgaria. Available from: https://www.mh.government.bg/media/filer_public/2016/06/07/zapoved-rd-01-193-03-06-2016-metodichesko-ukazanie-hiv-infekciq.pdf. [Accessed: 30 November 2018]

[23] Methodology Guidance on Prophylaxis of HIV Transmission from Mother to Child Available from: https://www.mh.government.bg/media/filer_public/2016/04/08/metodichesko_mtct_arv_zapoved_rd_01_83_17march2016_pechat.pdf. [Accessed: 30 November 2018]

[24] World health organization. Diet, Nutrition and Prevention of Chronic Diseases. Report of the joint WHO/FO expert consultation. Available from: https://www.who.int/dietphysicalactivity/publications/trs916/summary/en/. [Accessed: 01 December 2018]

[25] Kalichman SC, Cherry C, White D, Jones M, Koalichman MO, et al. Use of dietary supplements among people living with HIV/AIDS is associated with vulnerability to medical misinformation on the internet. AIDS Research and Therapy. 2012;**9**:1

[26] U.S. Department of Health and Human Services: HIV and Nutrition and Food Safety. Available from: https://aidsinfo.nih.gov/understanding-hiv-aids/fact-sheets/27/97/hiv-and-nutrition-and-food-safety. [Accessed: 01 December 2018]

[27] Canada's Source for HIV and Hepatitis C Information: A Practical Guide to Nutrition for People Living with HIV. Available from: https://www.catie.ca/en/practical-guides/nutrition. [Accessed: 01 December 2018]

[28] Nutrition and HIV: Available from: http://aidsbg.info/articleDisplay. aspx?aid=112. [Accessed: 01 December 2018]

[29] Galache JJ, Bailey R, Potischman N, Dwyer JT. Dietary supplement use was very high among older adults in the United States in 2011-2014. The Journal of Nutrition. 2017;**147**(1):1968-1976. DOI: https://doi.org/10.3945/jn.117.255984

[30] Stoimenova A. Food supplements in Central and Eastern European Countries. Acta Medica Bulgarica. 2010;**XXXVII**(1):71-77

Chapter 5

Basic Principles of Nutrition, HIV and AIDS: Making Improvements in Diet to Enhance Health

Ezinna E. Enwereji, Martina C. Ezeama and Prince E.N. Onyemachi

Abstract

The relationships among nutritional status, infectious diseases and immune system suggest nutrition as a cofactor in human immunodeficiency virus (HIV) progression. Poor nutritional status and HIV infection interact with each other leading to the development of opportunistic infections, malignancies, debilitation and death. Infection by human immunodeficiency virus (HIV) is characterized by progressive destruction of immune system. Malnutrition that is multifactorial is, therefore, one of the major complications of HIV infection that is poorly addressed in HIV intervention. Early nutritional intervention when individuals living with HIV show active weight loss is important in maximizing gain of lean body mass. Since malnutrition is the major complication of HIV infection, which results in wasting syndrome, it should be termed as a prognostic factor in advanced HIV infection though malnutrition is a result of not only HIV infection but also numerous HIV-associated complications. Studies have recommended clinical trials to evaluate prevalence of malnutrition among those living with HIV so as to examine the efficacy of supplementing with specific nutrients at various stages of HIV infection as well as combining therapeutic foods for treating malnutrition with antiretroviral treatment in children of HIV-positive mothers. Therefore, good nutrition guarantees excellent health in HIV infection.

Keywords: HIV, malnutrition, nutrition security, therapeutic foods, lipodystrophy, opportunistic infections

1. Introduction

Infants born to mothers living with HIV have poorer growth and higher morbidity and mortality than those born to mothers who are not infected with HIV. Furthermore, abnormalities in growth are common in children infected with HIV. Children living with HIV and AIDS are at increased risk of malnutrition. Chronic infections, especially HIV and AIDS, can lead to poor appetite and growth because food intake and nutrient absorption which the body needs in order to fight the infection are defective. The result is a weakened immune system that is ill equipped to fight the virus and other infections like tuberculosis. This accounts for the severe acute malnutrition seen in most people living with HIV. To increase the chances of survival of these people, therapeutic foods for reducing malnutrition should be combined with antiretroviral treatment to stop the infection from progressing [1, 2]. Studies indicate that multiple nutritional abnormalities occur relatively early in human immunodeficiency virus (HIV) infection, and also that decreased plasma levels of vitamins B6, B12, A, E and zinc are correlated with dietary intake and associated with significant alterations in immune response and cognitive function for people living with HIV infection. To determine the level of intake consistent with normal plasma nutrient levels, there is a need to examine nutrition status in relation to food consumption and nutrient supplementation in HIV seropositives [3, 4].

In developing countries where most families live in abject poverty and are exposed to infections due to poor nutrition and sanitation and contaminated drinking water, the benefits of HIV-positive mothers breastfeeding infants will greatly reduce the risk of HIV infection when ARVs are combined with good nutrition. In this instance, the nutrients and antibodies present in breast milk will make the healthiest food for such babies, thereby providing them with unmatched protections from HIV infection, diseases and even death. Therefore, good nutrition will lay the foundation for healthy thriving and productivity of people living with HIV. Now more than ever, there is global recognition that good nutrition is the key to sustainable development. But good nutrition is more than about just ending hunger: it is also crucial to achieving some targets, including ending poverty, achieving gender equality, ensuring healthy lives, promoting lifelong learning, improving economic growth, building inclusive societies and ensuring sustainable consumption [5–7]. Nutritional status may have an impact at all stages of HIV disease since most of the clinical features of HIV infection originate from nutritional problems which are exacerbated by the presence of malnutrition. However, inadequate food intake, due to a variety of etiologies, malabsorption and altered metabolism, may also contribute to malnutrition. Additionally, factors in food, including reduced micronutrient levels, can negatively affect the immune functions and result in increase in the progression of HIV infection at all stages [8–11].

The frequent weight loss in people living with HIV worsens the prognosis of the infection. Their reduced dietary intake, increased digestive problems and energy expenditure result in severe malnutrition. Therefore, the nutritional support and its association with anabolic agents to promote tissue growth and physical activity should be carefully selected [12–14]. The adverse effects of some new antiretroviral drugs could influence the patients' nutritional state as well as compliance to treatments. In cases where lipodystrophy, whose etiology is still unknown and no treatment has yet been found, and metabolic disorders like dyslipidemia, glucose intolerance and others occur, particular attention should be given since these conditions are likely to increase cardiovascular risks and, moreover, they are generally sensitive to a dietary approach [2, 15, 16].

Achieving and maintaining optimal nutrition is considered an important strategy for ensuring food security for people infected with HIV. A good nutrition can improve an individual's immune function, limit disease complications, and improve quality of life and survival. This is necessary because macronutrient interventions, such as balanced diet of high protein, high carbohydrate and high fat, will reduce morbidity and mortality of people living with HIV infection. Evidence has shown that macronutrient supplementation will reduce HIV-related complications, such as opportunistic infections or death. Food insecurity has been recognized as the key driver of HIV epidemic and a potential cause of poor health outcomes among people living with HIV and AIDS. Food insecurity is linked with heart disease, diabetes, obesity, depression and is independently associated with incomplete HIV RNA suppression among HIV-infected individuals [17]. These call for holistic and comprehensive response in minimizing chronic nutrition insecurity among HIV-positive persons. Therefore, the need to elucidate ways of sustaining long-term nutritional support for HIV-positive individuals to minimize nutritional insecurity and guarantee security in livelihood should not be underestimated.

2. The foundations of good nutrition

Nutrition is defined as the sum total of the processes by which a living organism receives materials from its environment and uses them to promote its own vital activities. The materials which it receives are known as nutrients. Nutrition is also the science that interprets the relationship between the food consumed and its function on the living organism. It relates to food intake and functions in the body for the overall well-being of the individual. It includes the intake of food, liberation of energy, elimination of waste and all the synthesis or processes that are essential for the maintenance of growth and reproduction of the individual [18]. The relationship between nutrition and HIV is a vicious cycle, similar to the relationship between nutrition and other infections. Compromises in nutritional status and poor nutrition further weaken the immune system and thereby increase susceptibility to opportunistic infections. Poor nutrition increases the body's vulnerability to infections, and infections aggravate poor nutrition. Inadequate dietary intake leads to poor nutrition and lowers immune system functioning. Poor nutrition reduces the body's ability to fight infections and therefore helps increase the incidence, severity and length of infections. Research has shown that clinically, there are synergistic interactions between infection, nutritional status and immune functions. Infectious diseases, no matter how mild, will influence nutritional status and conversely cause nutrient deficiencies that are sufficiently severe to impair resistance to infection [19, 20].

The foundations of good nutrition include improving women's nutrition before, during and after pregnancy; promoting and supporting exclusive breastfeeding for the first 6 months of a child's life, and continued breastfeeding up to age 2 or beyond; providing timely, safe, appropriate and high-quality complementary foods as well as micronutrient interventions. In this regard, nutritional status should be assessed using biochemical measurement of nutrient levels, dietary history, anthropometry and clinical examination for the signs and symptoms of nutritional deficiency or excess. In managing emergencies, UNICEF's programs have concentrated their interventions on foundations of good nutrition, prevention and treatment of malnutrition to vulnerable groups including those living with HIV and AIDS irrespective of whether or not they are using highly active antiretroviral therapy (HAART) which has been postulated to reduce the occurrence of human immunodeficiency virus (HIV)-associated weight loss and wasting. To this assumption, studies have shown that there is no difference in the extent of wasting experienced between those who received HAART and those who did not. It has been shown that the weight loss or wasting in HIV infection can be radically reduced with nutrition intervention. The good news is that the goal of nutritional intervention is usually to preserve lean body mass and provide adequate nutrients as well as minimize symptoms of malabsorption and thereby improve quality of life. This is why specific nutritional therapy ranges from oral supplements to home total parenteral nutrition (TPN) which is individualized [21, 22].

Following interventions proffered by several organizations and researchers to reduce malnutrition among persons living with HIV, the definition of wasting developed by the Centers for Disease Control and Prevention (CDC) in 1987 has been adopted by researchers. This definition requires an involuntary weight loss of >10% of baseline body weight plus diarrhea, fever, or weakness for >30 days to be termed as wasting. Most researchers have now dropped the comorbid conditions of wasting and have simply espoused weight loss >10% as the definition of HIV-associated wasting. In the CDC definition, "baseline weight" is neither defined nor time frame specified for the weight loss. Presently, most researchers are using the definition of wasting as that which will require a weight loss >5% in a 6-month period and that in which the weight loss is sustained. Some other studies have shown that this level of weight loss can predict mortality and infectious complications in individuals with AIDS and that reduction in a body mass index to <20 kg/m^2 in a 6-month period should be used as an index of wasting among HIV and AIDS clients when intervening for malnutrition. Because of the uncertainty as to which of these definitions given above should be adopted as the standard definition of wasting for intervention, the three presented criteria are now being used. Therefore, weight loss and wasting continue to be common problems for individuals infected with HIV as well as for those treated with HAART in whom either HAART has failed or there is lack of tolerance for HAART regimens [23, 24].

Studies have been done to determine whether specific nutrient abnormalities occur in earlier stages of HIV infection, thereby preceding the marked wasting and malnutrition that accompany later stages of the infection. It has been found that even as life expectancy increases with antiretroviral therapy (ART), age-related comorbidities now contribute to the main burden of disease associated with HIV infection. These comorbidities have been reported to occur regularly among HIV-infected individuals, thereby resulting in conditions associated with nutritional deficiencies that are typically seen in the elderly and in middle-aged HIV-infected individuals. This suggests that age decline occurs independent of chronological age in the HIV-infected individuals. These observations have led to the conclusion that HIV infection accelerates the biological aging process. Therefore, aging in HIV infection is a multifactorial process involving complex interplay of biological and non-biological constructs which may differ depending on the socioeconomic and nutritional statuses of HIV individuals. The prolonged nutritional deficiencies with chronic coinfections and exposures to more toxic antiretroviral drugs constitute risks to people living with HIV and AIDS [24]. However, evidence has shown that patients who enrolled in food supplement intervention while on treatment regimens self-reported greater adherence to their medications, fewer side effects, increased weight gain, recovery of physical strength and the resumption of labor activities. Therefore, promoting sound feeding practices is one of the strategies to ensure good health for people living positively with HIV and AIDS.

2.1 Nutrition for sustainable development

Ideally, good nutrition lays the foundation for healthy and productive environments for people living positively with HIV infection. Well-nourished HIV individuals are more resistant to diseases and crises, and can perform their daily duties better than those that are poorly nourished. This shows that well-nourished HIV persons are better able to participate in and contribute to the development of their communities. Therefore, the benefits of good nutrition for people living positively with HIV act as the "glue" binding together and supporting their contributions to various facets of a nation's development, especially now that there is a global recognition that good nutrition is the key to sustainable development. Specifically, the objective of Goal 2 of the 2015 Sustainable Development Goals (SDGs) aims to "end hunger, achieve food security, improve nutrition, and sustainable agriculture" and thereby promote good health. Therefore, good nutrition is more than just about ending hunger: it also includes achieving many SDG targets, such as ending poverty, achieving gender equality, ensuring healthy lives, promoting lifelong learning, improving economic growth, building inclusive societies and guaranteeing sustainable consumption of quality foods. This will reduce inequalities among persons living with HIV and make sure that guidelines on appropriate feeding are available to all, including those with limited access to health care services. Convinced that it is now time for governments in developing countries to renew their commitment to protect and promote optimal feeding that will guarantee good health for persons living with HIV and AIDS.

The level of total intake (diet plus supplements) for all nutrients that would guarantee optimal health for persons living with HIV should be clearly emphasized to achieve normal plasma nutrient values since persons living with HIV and AIDS appear to require nutrient intake in multiples of the recommended dietary allowance (RDA) for vitamins A, E, B6, B12, iron, zinc and others. Therefore, effective program for nutritional supplements may be beneficial in maintaining adequate plasma nutrient levels for persons living with HIV and AIDS. This means that the biochemical measurements of nutrient status, dietary history, anthropometry, clinical signs or symptoms that will show nutritional excesses or deficiencies among persons living with HIV and AIDS should be regularly done to ascertain their health statuses since provision of nutritional supplements acts as an adjunct to ART. Though studies have identified the fear of persons living with HIV developing too much appetite but not having enough to eat as the major obstacle to their non-acceptance of nutritional supplements, it should be emphasized that this obstacle should not preclude the provision of adequate dietary supplements to improve both adherence and prognosis to those living positively with HIV and AIDS [25, 26]. Therefore, the need to increase and integrate nutritional supplements into ART programs to improve adherence and maximize the benefits of therapy should not be underestimated.

This means that the principles of healthy eating for HIV-positive persons to ensure sustainable development will require that all the necessary food nutrients are added in the daily meals and in the right proportions. Therefore, meals that will guarantee optimal health for HIV-positive persons should include:

- a diet high in vegetables, fruits, whole grains and legumes

- lean and low-fat sources of protein

- limited sweets, soft drinks and foods with added sugar

- proteins, carbohydrates and a little good fat in all meals and snacks

Specifically, the HIV-positive individuals should be encouraged to add foods rich in calories. Foods rich in calories will provide the body with fuel to maintain lean body mass. To get enough calories, they need to consume the following in these proportions:

- 17 calories per pound of the body weight so as to maintain body weight

- 20 calories per pound of the body weight if an opportunistic infection has occurred

- 25 calories per pound if there is loss of body weight

Protein will help to build the muscles and organs and guarantee strong immune system for HIV-positive persons and should be consumed in enough quantity. To get the right proportion and types of protein, HIV-positive persons should aim at having these in the diet:

- 100–150 grams a day, if an HIV-positive man

- 80–100 grams a day, if an HIV-positive woman

- If there is kidney problem, more than 15–20% of the calories from protein should not be consumed. This is because too much of such calories will put stress on the kidney and thereby compromise kidney function.

Also, lean meat such as pork, beef, skinless chicken, fish and low-fat dairy products should be consumed. To get extra protein, there is need to add vegetable proteins such as legumes, nuts, vegetables and others. For carbohydrates which will give energy, HIV-positive persons should eat the right types and proportions of carbohydrates by:

• Eating five to six servings of fruits and vegetables each day.

• Adding to the meals fruits with a variety of colors so as to get a wide range of nutrients.

• Eating legumes and whole grains, such as brown rice, corn and others. However, if HIV individuals do not have gluten sensitivity, whole-wheat flour, oats and barley may be good enough for them. But if there is gluten sensitivity, whole-wheat flour should not be taken. Then, brown rice and potato should form useful sources of carbohydrate. If HIV individuals are diabetic or pre-diabetic or have insulin resistance, most of their carbohydrates should come from vegetables.

• The practice of consuming much of simple sugars, such as candy, cake, cookies and ice cream should be limited for HIV-positive persons.

Fat will provide extra energy. For HIV-positive persons to get enough of the right kinds of fat for energy, the following should be observed:

• 10% or more of daily calories should come from monounsaturated fats like nuts, seeds, avocado, fish, canola and olive oils.

• less than 10% of daily calories should be made up of polyunsaturated fats such as fish, walnuts, flax seed, corn, sunflower, soybean and safflower oil.

• less than 7% of daily calories should be saturated fats like fatty meat, poultry with skin, butter, whole-milk dairy foods, coconut and palm oils.

• 30% of daily calories should come from fat like omega-3 fatty acid.

Omega-3 fatty acids are essential fats that must be present in the diet of HIV-positive individuals. Consuming these healthy fats that the body cannot produce unlike other fats has important benefits for the HIV persons' body and brain. However, most HIV-positive people whose meals are mainly made up of standard Western diet end up not eating enough omega-3 fats. Omega-3 fatty acids are polyunsaturated fats that the body needs but cannot produce on its own. For this reason, omega-3 fatty acids are classified as essential fatty acids. There are basically three important types of omega-3 fatty acids that are beneficial to the health of HIV-positive individuals. The first is eicosapentaenoic acid (EPA). This is a 20-carbon-long chain omega-3 fatty acid, primarily found in fatty fish, seafood and fish oils. EPA is important in the formation of signaling molecules like eicosanoids that will reduce inflammation. EPA is effective in protecting HIV persons against depression. The second type of omega-3 is docosahexaenoic acid (DHA). DHA is a 22-carbon-long chain omega-3 fatty acid primarily found in fatty fish, seafood, fish oils and algae. The main role of DHA is to serve as a structural component in cell membranes, particularly in the nerve cells of the brain and eyes. DHA constitutes about 40% of the polyunsaturated fats in the brain. DHA is very important during pregnancy and breastfeeding. It helps in the development of the nervous system of the fetus. Breast milk contains significant amounts of DHA. The third type of omega-3 is alpha-linolenic acid (ALA), an 18-carbon-long chain omega-3 fatty acid found in high-fat plant foods like flax seeds, cotton seed, walnuts and others. Though it is the most common omega-3 fatty acid found in the diet, it is not very active in the body. ALA needs to be converted to EPA and DHA before it can be active. Unfortunately, only about 5% of ALA gets converted to EPA and as little as 0.5% will be converted to DHA. For this reason, HIV-positive persons' consumption of omega-3 fatty acids should consist mainly of EPA and DHA than ALA. Most of the ALA eaten is simply used for energy [27–29].

2.1.1 Health effects of omega-3 fats

Omega-3 fatty acids have both negative and positive effects when consumed in certain proportions. On the positive side, omega-3 fatty acids have several health benefits in various body systems. For example, studies have shown that omega-3 supplements will significantly lower blood triglycerides. Consuming foods such as salmon, sardines, cod liver oil and others that contain enough amounts of omega-3 has been linked to reduced risk of colon, prostrate and breast cancers. Taking omega-3 fatty acid supplement helps to reduce excess fat in the liver. Consuming omega-3 supplements like fish oil helps to reduce symptoms of depression and anxiety. Inflammation, pain and other symptoms of autoimmune diseases such as in rheumatoid arthritis have been reduced using omega-3 supplements. Omega-3 has been found effective in controlling menstrual pains and in preventing asthma in children and young adults. DHA if taken during pregnancy and breastfeeding has been found to improve the intellectual and eye development of the child. Studies have linked a higher intake of omega-3 to a reduced risk of Alzheimer's disease and dementia. However, for optimal health, mainstream health organizations like the World Health Organization and European Food Safety Authority recommend a minimum of 250–500 mg combined EPA and DHA each day for healthy adults. The American Heart Association recommends eating fatty fish at least two times per week in order to ensure optimal omega-3 intake for heart disease prevention. For pregnant and breastfeeding women, it is recommended to add an additional 200 mg of DHA to the recommended intake.

On the negative side, consuming more than the upper limit of omega-3 fatty acid will have adverse health effects. According to food and drug agencies (FDA), taking up to 2000 mg of combined EPA and DHA per day from supplements will be safe, but in high doses, omega-3 fatty acids can cause blood thinning and excessive bleeding. Therefore, care should be taken in the consumption of omega-3 if an individual has a bleeding disorder or is taking blood-thinning medications. It has been shown that some omega-3 supplements, especially fish oil, can cause digestive problems and unpleasant fish oil burps because many omega-3 supplements are high in calories. For example, cod liver oil is very high in vitamin A, and can be harmful when taken in large doses. The bottom line is that taking up to 2000 mg of omega-3 per day from supplements is safe according to the FDA, but anything more than this is classified as lethal. The fact remains that getting enough omega-3 fatty acid is not difficult when one eats fishes. For instance, when one consumes salmon, one gets 4023 mg per serving (EPA and DHA). For cod liver oil, one gets 2664 mg per serving (EPA and DHA); for sardines, 2205 mg per serving (EPA and DHA); for anchovies, one gets 2338 mg of ALA per serving; for chia seeds or cotton seeds, one gets 2338 mg of ALA per serving; and for walnuts, 2542 mg of ALA per serving. Consuming other foods that are high in EPA and DHA such as fatty fish, meat, eggs and dairy products from grass-fed or pasture-raised animals and other common plant foods high in the ALA such as soya beans, hemp seeds, walnuts, spinach and Brussels sprouts can be deleterious to health. However, excess omega-3 in the body will be used as a source of energy like other fats. Assuming HIV-positive individuals have no opportunity of eating fatty fish or seafood, taking omega-3 supplement to improve both physical and mental health as well as reduce the risk of disease infections should be seriously considered [30–32].

2.2 Vitamins and minerals

Vitamins and minerals regulate body processes and so people who are HIV-positive need extra vitamins and minerals in the diet to repair and heal damaged cells. They need extra vitamins and minerals to boost the immune system. These vitamins and minerals which should be added in the diet include:

- Vitamin A and beta-carotene, from dark green, yellow, orange, or red vegetables and fruits including liver, whole eggs, and milk

- Vitamin B, from meat, fish, chicken, grains, nuts, white beans, avocados, broccoli and green leafy vegetables

- Vitamin C, from citrus fruits

- Vitamin E, from green leafy vegetables, peanuts and vegetable oils

- Selenium, from whole grains, nuts, poultry, fish, eggs and peanut butter

- Zinc, from meat, poultry, fish, beans, peanuts, and milk and other dairy products

Because of the difficulty for HIV-positive persons in getting enough of all the nutrients needed for optimal health from foods, it is recommended that a multivitamin/mineral tablet (without extra iron) but containing 100% of the recommended daily allowance (RDA) should be taken. If at least three servings of high-calcium food such as green leafy vegetables or dairy foods are not eaten on daily basis, calcium supplements could be taken in the diet.

2.2.1 Nutrition and HIV: coping with special problems

HIV-positive persons could have a variety of reactions including side effects from ART medications which should be managed. Here are some of the problems that HIV persons need to control:

Nausea and vomiting:
To manage nausea and vomiting, they need to:

- Eat bland, low-fat foods, such as plain pasta, canned fruit, or plain broth.

- Eat smaller meals every 1–2 hours.

- Avoid greasy or spicy foods, or foods with strong odors.

- Drink ginger tea or ginger ale or ginger.

- Eat more cold foods and less hot foods.

- Rest after meals, but not to lie down flat.

- Receive medications for nausea.

Diarrhea: for diarrhea, they need to:

- Drink more fluids than usual including diluted juices.

- Limit taking milk, sugary or caffeinated drinks.

- Eat slowly and more frequently.

- Avoid greasy foods.

- Add briefly in the diet bananas, rice, apple sauce and toast (B.R.A.T).

- Avoid eating uncooked foods including vegetables but rather eat well-cooked ones.

- Take calcium carbonate supplements or fiber supplements such as wafers.

Lack of appetite: for lack of appetite they need to:

- Add ginger in the diet to help stimulate appetite and improve digestion.

- Avoid drinking too much fluid before meals.

- Make meals as attractive as possible.

- Take smaller but frequent meals.

- Add foods rich in antioxidants such as ginger, cranberries, raspberries, blackberries, walnuts and others.

- Take medications that will stimulate appetite.

Too much weight loss: for this, HIV-positive persons should:

- Include enough protein, carbohydrates and fats in the diet.

- Increase the intake of dietary iron foods such as lean red meat, chicken, fish, beans, lentils, cashew, spinach, whole-grain bread and others to reduce anemia.

- Eat vitamin C-rich foods during meals to increase the absorption of non-heme iron.

- Take cereals and add ice cream to desserts.

- Eat dried fruits or nuts for snacks.

- Add nutrition supplements, such as boost, carnation instant and others in the breakfast.

- Take medications that stimulate appetite and also treat nausea.

Mouth and swallowing problems: these can be controlled by:

- Eating only soft foods such as yogurt, mashed potatoes, or rice.

- Not eating raw vegetables.

- Eating softer fruits, such as bananas or pears.

- Avoiding acidic foods, such as oranges, lemons and tomatoes.

- Visiting a doctor to rule out opportunistic infections.

Lipodystrophy (fat redistribution syndrome): this can be controlled by:

- Avoiding saturated and transfats in the diet.

- Taking unsaturated fats and sources of omega-3 fatty acids, such as salmon and tuna.

- Restricting the consumption of alcohol, and refined sugars.

- Preventing insulin resistance by avoiding foods that can raise glucose and insulin levels, primarily the carbohydrates.

- Eating fiber-rich whole grains, fruits and vegetables.

Even in the absence of opportunistic infections, many people with HIV infection may experience these health problems; therefore, the relationships between health problems and nutritional status of HIV-positive persons must be addressed to achieve the benefits of optimum health [14, 33].

3. Conclusion

Malnutrition can be used as a measure of food insecurity and HIV individuals with compromised immune system will be at risk of infections when malnourished. HIV infection leads to many nutritional problems. Conditions such as malnutrition and opportunistic infections exacerbate HIV infection. The increased caloric requirements of HIV-positive individuals, the undesirable side effects of treatment that may be worsened by malnutrition, and the declines in adherence and possible drug resistance are justifications for strengthening the nutrition security of HIV-positive individuals including those receiving antiretroviral treatment.

For a long time, the wasting syndrome has been the most frequently reported feature of HIV and AIDS. Nutritional and micronutrient deficiencies play important role in immune degradation and impaired development in HIV infection. Proper nutrition complemented by careful implementation of antiretroviral drugs is essential in the response to HIV and AIDS pandemic. Realizing the value of nutrition to the health of people living positively with HIV and AIDS, especially those suffering from severe acute malnutrition, UNICEF supports them with therapeutic feeding and antiretroviral therapy. That is, UNICEF provides support for nutritional assessments and counseling to manage HIV infection and the side effects of antiretroviral drugs. Therefore, body wasting, characterized by loss of body cell mass, which is frequently experienced by people with HIV infection and a factor in survival itself can be reduced by UNICEF's intervention and thereby minimize rapid weight loss typically associated with episodes of secondary infections. Therefore, adequate nutrition is a panacea for the good health of HIV persons.

Basic Principles of Nutrition, HIV and AIDS: Making Improvements in Diet to Enhance Health
DOI: http://dx.doi.org/10.5772/intechopen.84719

Author details

Ezinna E. Enwereji[1*], Martina C. Ezeama[2] and Prince E.N. Onyemachi[1]

1 Abia State University, Nigeria

2 Imo State University, Owerri, Nigeria

*Address all correspondence to: hersng@yahoo.com

IntechOpen

References

[1] UNGASS (United Nations General Assembly Special Session on HIV/AIDS). Article 28 in Declaration of Commitment by the United Nations General Assembly Special Session Dedicated to HIV/AIDS. New York: United Nations. 2006. Available from: http://www.ungass.org

[2] Semba RD, Tang AM. Micronutrients and the pathogenesis of human immunodeficiency virus infection. The British Journal of Nutrition. 1999;**81**:181-189

[3] World Health Organization. Nutrient Requirements for People Living with HIV/AIDS: Report of a Technical Consultation. Geneva: WHO; 2003

[4] Mangili A, Murman DH, Zampini AM, Wanke CA. Nutrition and HIV infection: Review of weight loss and wasting in the era of highly active antiretroviral therapy from the nutrition and healthy living cohort. Clinical Infectious Diseases. 2006;**42**:836-842

[5] Laurent C, Ngom Gueye NF, Ndour CT, Gueye PM, Diouf M, Diakhate N, et al. Long-term benefits of highly active antiretroviral therapy in Senegalese HIV-1-infected adults. Journal of Acquired Immune Deficiency Syndromes. 2005;**38**:14-17

[6] Miller CJ, Baker JV, Bormann AM, Erlandson KM, Huppler Hullsiek K, Justice AC, et al. Adjudicated morbidity and mortality outcomes by age among individuals with HIV infection on suppressive antiretroviral therapy. PLoS One. 2014;**9**:e95061

[7] Guaraldi G, Orlando G, Zona S, Menozzi M, Carli F, Garlassi E, et al. Premature age-related comorbidities among HIV-infected persons compared with the general population. Clinical Infectious Diseases. 2011;**53**:1120-1126

[8] Pathai S, Gilbert C, Weiss HA, Cook C, Wood R, Bekker LG, et al. Frailty in HIV-infected adults in South Africa. Journal of Acquired Immune Deficiency Syndromes. 2013;**62**:43-51

[9] Levett TJ, Cresswell FV, Malik MA, Fisher M, Wright J. Systematic review of prevalence and predictors of frailty in individuals with human immunodeficiency virus. Journal of the American Geriatrics Society. 2016;**64**:1006-1014

[10] Erlandson KM, Allshouse AA, Rapaport E, Palmer BE, Wilson CC, Weinberg A, et al. Physical function impairment of older, HIV-infected adults is associated with cytomegalovirus immunoglobulin response. AIDS Research and Human Retroviruses. 2015;**31**:905-912

[11] Dannhauser A, van Staden AM, van der Ryst E, et al. Nutritional status of HIV-1 seropositive patients in Free State Province of South Africa: Anthropometric and dietary profile. European Journal of Clinical Nutrition. 1999;**53**:165-173

[12] Stolbach A, Paziana K, Heverling H, Pham P. A review of the toxicity of HIV edications II: Interactions with drugs and complementary and alternative medicine products. Journal of Medical Toxicology. 2015;**11**:326-341

[13] Niyongabo T, Henzel D, Ndayishimyie JM, et al. Nutritional status of adult inpatients in Bujumbura, Burundi (impact of HIV infection). European Journal of Clinical Nutrition. 1999;**53**:579-582

[14] Castetbon K, Kadio A, Bondurand A, et al. Nutritional status and dietary intakes in human immunodeficiency virus (HIV)-infected outpatients in Abidjan, Côte D'Ivoire, 1995. European Journal of Clinical Nutrition. 1997;**51**:81-86

[15] Ehrenpreis ED, Carlson SJ, Boorstein HL, et al. Malabsorption and deficiency of vitamin B12 in HIV-infected patients with chronic diarrhea. Digestive Diseases and Sciences. 1994;39:2159-2162

[16] Koch J, Neal EA, Schlott MJ, et al. Zinc levels and infections in hospitalized patients with HIV/AIDS. Nutrition. 1996;12:515-518

[17] Allard JP, Aghdassi E, Chau J, et al. Oxidative stress and plasma antioxidant micronutrients in humans with HIV infection. The American Journal of Clinical Nutrition. 1998;67:143-147

[18] Dudgeon WD, Phillips KD, Carson JA, Brewer RB, Durstine JL, Hand GA. Counteracting muscle wasting in HIV-infected individuals. HIV Medicine. 2006;7:299-310. DOI: 10.1111/j.1468-1293.2006.00380.x

[19] Mastroiacovo P, Ajassa C, Berardelli G, et al. Antioxidant vitamins and immunodeficiency. International Journal for Vitamin and Nutrition Research. 1996;66:141-145

[20] Look MP, Rockstroh JK, Rao GS, et al. Serum selenium, plasma glutathione (GSH) and erythrocyte glutathione peroxidase (GSH-Px)-levels in asymptomatic versus symptomatic human immunodeficiency virus-1 (HIV-1) infection. European Journal of Clinical Nutrition. 1997;51:266-272

[21] Semba RD, Kumwenda N, Hoover DR, et al. Assessment of iron status using plasma transferrin receptor in pregnant women with and without human immunodeficiency virus infection in Malawi. European Journal of Clinical Nutrition. 2000;54:872-877

[22] Antelman G, Msamanga GI, Spiegelman D, et al. Nutritional factors and infectious disease contribute to anemia among pregnant women with Human Immunodeficiency Virus in

Tanzania. The Journal of Nutrition. 2000;130:1950-1957

[23] Falutz J, Tsoukas C, Gold P. Zinc as a cofactor in human immunodeficiency virus-induced immuno-suppression. Journal of the American Medical Association. 1998;259:2850-2851

[24] Clark RH, Feleke G, Din M, et al. Nutritional treatment for acquired immunodeficiency virus-associated wasting using beta-hydroxy beta-methylbutyrate, glutamine, and arginine: A randomized, double-blind, placebo-controlled study. Journal of Parenteral and Enteral Nutrition. 2000;24:133-139

[25] Baum MK, Shor-Posner G, Zhang G, et al. HIV-1 infection in women is associated with severe nutritional deficiencies. Journal of Acquired Immune Deficiency Syndromes and Human Retrovirology. 1997;16:272-278

[26] Wheeler DA, Gilbert CL, Launer CA, et al. Weight loss as a predictor of survival and disease progression in HIV infection. Terry Beirn community programs for clinical research on AIDS. Journal of Acquired Immune Deficiency Syndromes and Human Retrovirology. 1998;18:80-85

[27] Melchior JC, Niyongabo T, Henzel D, et al. Malnutrition and wasting, immunodeficiency, and chronic inflammation as independent predictors of survival in HIV-infected patients. Nutrition. 1999;15:865-869

[28] Gibert CL, Wheeler DA, Collins G, et al. Randomized, controlled trial of caloric supplements in HIV infection. Terry Beirn community programs for clinical research on AIDS. Journal of Acquired Immune Deficiency Syndromes. 1999;22:253-259

[29] Bogden JD, Kemp FW, Han S, et al. Status of selected nutrients and progression of human

immunodeficiency virus type 1
infection. The American Journal of
Clinical Nutrition. 2000;**72**:809-815

[30] Coutsoudis A, Moodley D,
Pillay K, et al. Effects of vitamin A
supplementation on viral load in
HIV-1-infected pregnant women.
Journal of Acquired Immune Deficiency
Syndromes and Human Retrovirology.
1997;**15**:86-87

[31] Kelly P, Musonda R, Kafwembe E,
et al. Micronutrient supplementation in
the AIDS diarrhoea wasting syndrome
in Zambia: A randomized controlled
trial. AIDS. 1999;**13**:495-500

[32] Au JT, Kayitenkore K, Shutes E,
et al. Access to adequate nutrition is a
major potential obstacle to antiretroviral
adherence among HIV-infected
individuals in Rwanda. AIDS Journal.
2006;**20**(16):2116-2118

[33] Erlandson KM, Allshouse AA,
Jankowski CM, Mawhinney S, Kohrt
WM, Campbell TB. Relationship
of physical function and quality
of life among persons aging with
HIV infection. AIDS Journal.
2014;**28**:1939-1943

www.ingramcontent.com/pod-product-compliance
Lightning Source LLC
Chambersburg PA
CBHW081238190326
41458CB00016B/5835